BRADY

EMT-Basic National Standards Review Self Test

C.D. Miller, REMT-P
David White

Based on the
Emergency Medical Technician
National Standard Curriculum
U. S. Department of Transportation,
National Highway Traffic Safety Administration

Keyed to
Brady's *Emergency Care*
5th Edition, © 1990

BRADY
PRENTICE HALL CAREER & TECHNOLOGY
Englewood Cliffs, New Jersey 07632

Library of Congress Cataloging-in-Publication Data

Miller . C. D. (Charly D.), (date)
    EMT-basic national standards review self test / by C.D. Miller,
David White.
        p.   cm.
    "Based on the Emergency medical technician national standard
curriculum [by] U.S. Department of Transportation, National Highway
Traffic Safety Administration."
    "Keyed to Brady's emergency care, fifth edition, 1990."
    ISBN 0-89303-875-X
    1. Emergency medicine—Examinations, questions, etc.   2. First aid
in illness and injury—Examinations, questions, etc.   3. Rescue
work—Examinations, questions etc.   4. Emergency medical personnel—
Examinations, questions, etc.   I. White, David, (date) .
II. Grant, Harvey D., (date) Brady emergency care.   III. United
States. National Highway Safety Administration.   IV. Title.
    [DNLM: 1. Emergencies—Examination questions.   2. Emergency
Medical Services—United States.   3. Emergency Medical Technicians—
examination questions.   WB 18 M647e]
RC86.7.G7   1990 Suppl.
616.02'2—dc20
DNLM/DLC   92-8068
for Library of Congress   CIP

Acquisitions Editor: **Natalie Anderson**
Editorial Assistant: **Louise Fullam**
Cover Designer: **Marianne Frasco**
Interior Design and Layout: **Lightworks Design**
Prepress Buyer: **Ilene Levy**
Manufacturing Buyer: **Ed O'Dougherty**

 ©1992 by Prentice Hall Career & Technology
Prentice-Hall, Inc.
A Paramount Communications Company
Englewood Cliffs, New Jersey 07632

Printed in the United States of America
10 9 8 7 6 5 4

ISBN 0-89303-875-X

Prentice-Hall International (UK) Limited, *London*
Prentice-Hall of Australia Pty. Limited, *Sydney*
Prentice-Hall Canada Inc., *Toronto*
Prentice-Hall Hispanoamericana, S.A., *Mexico*
Prentice-Hall of India Private Limited, *New Delhi*
Prentice-Hall of Japan, Inc., *Tokyo*
Simon & Schuster Asia Pte. Ltd., *Singapore*
Editora Prentice-Hall do Brasil, Ltda., *Rio de Janeiro*

Contents

TEST SECTION ONE 1

Roles and Responsibilities; EMS Terminology; Medical Ethics; Legal Aspects of EMS; Extrication and Rescue; Communications; Ambulance Operations; Anatomy and Physiology; Patient Assessment; Medical Terminology.

TEST SECTION TWO 29

Airway Mechanics and Obstruction; Airway Adjuncts and Oxygen Delivery Systems; Respiratory Arrest and Resuscitation; Circulation; Cardiac Arrest and CPR; Poisons/Bites/Stings; Heart Attack; Stroke; Dyspnea; Medical Terminology.

TEST SECTION THREE 89

Diabetes; Convulsions; Acute Abdomen; Communicable Diseases; Substance Abuse; Pediatric Patients; Bleeding and Shock; Vital Signs; Anti-Shock Garments (PASG or MAST); Soft-Tissue Injuries; Fractures and Dislocations of the Upper and Lower Extremities; Heat Injuries; Hypothermia and Frostbite; Water-Related Injuries; Medical Terminology.

TEST SECTION FOUR **143**

Injuries to the Head, Face, Eyes, Neck, and Spine; Injuries to the Chest, Abdomen, and Genitalia; Emergency Childbirth; Burns (Thermal, Chemical, Electrical, Radiation); Hazardous Materials; Psychological Aspects of Emergency Care; Medical Terminology.

APPENDIX

Preface

Dear Reader,

This text is designed to assist you, the EMT-Basic, in your preparation for any written examination. It is based on the EMT National Standard Curriculum as set forth by the National Highway Traffic Safety Administration's Department of Transportation (DOT). Its self-test format is designed to challenge you, to pinpoint the subjects in which you require additional study, and to test your skill at reading and responding to test questions.

The answer keys are accompanied by subject title and reference page numbers that correspond to Brady's *Emergency Care*, 5th Edition. If you don't have that text (and cannot purchase it,) use the index of the text you do have to seek out information on the subjects you had difficulty with. Each section has questions on medical terminology. The answer key for some of these questions will direct you to reference your text glossary or a medical dictionary.

Although these tests cannot possibly guarantee you a perfect score, if you can pass the self-tests with 90 percent or better you should be able to achieve a similar score on any written exam you may face.

Be sure to read the sections we have included that provide tips on mental and physical preparation for taking written and practical exams. All too frequently, students fail tests *not because they don't know the material*, but because they don't read carefully or are ill-prepared to successfully perform in the testing environment.

We hope this text will assist you to excel in your examination. We do not wish you good luck, because luck is not a factor. Your dedicated preparation and review will help you to achieve high scores.

Sincerely yours,

C. D. Miller and David White

Acknowledgments

The authors wish to express their gratitude and appreciation to Natalie Anderson for making our children her children, and then encouraging us to have more!

Special thanks to Ann Shimkus for her contributions to this effort.

Additional thank-yous to Mike Keller and Bruce Adams.

Lastly, "Hi, Mom! Hi, Dad!" (Raymond and Carol Miller, James and Carolyn White).

About The Authors

Charly D. Miller is a paramedic, currently employed by Denver General Hospital's Paramedic Division. She has been involved in EMS since 1983, when she received her EMT-Basic certificate in the state of Nebraska. In addition to "working the streets," she has been an in-hospital Psychiatric Technician-EMT and a helicopter medic for the Army National Guard. She continues to work as a CPR instructor, an EMT and paramedic instructor, a faculty member for PHTLS and Critical Trauma Care workshops, an ACLS instructor, and a professional moulage artist. She received her paramedic training at Creighton University in Omaha, Nebraska and has been a Nationally Registered EMT-Paramedic since 1986. Her first Brady book, *Home Meds; A Paramedic's Pocket Guide To Prescription Medications* was published in the fall of 1991.

David White began his EMS career in 1985 as a firefighter EMT in Sheridan, Colorado. In 1986 he was certified at the EMT/IV level and began working for a private ambulance service in Cheyenne, Wyoming. He received his paramedic training in 1989 and is currently enrolled in a registered nursing program in Denver, Colorado.

Suggestions for Written Examination Preparation and Execution

Written examinations are generally as delightful as a visit to the dentist. However, anesthesia is an inappropriate solution.

Test preparation should start well before the exam day. Use this text to determine your strengths and weaknesses, and to practice your test-taking skills.

First, read each question carefully. Many written examinations are failed by knowledgeable and experienced EMTs *simply because they don't read the question well.* Don't read more into the question than what is presented. Is the question asking you to identify a correct answer, an incorrect answer, or the "best" answer? Read each answer carefully. After making your selection, go back and reread the question, inserting that answer. Does it still seem correct?

In an exam situation, a guess is better than leaving the answer completely blank (a blank answer is an error). When taking the self tests, however, *do not guess* at the answers. If you cannot answer a question with confidence, you ought to review that particular subject. If you *do* guess, you may answer correctly by pure accident. There is no guarantee that you will guess in the same manner when faced with a similar question on your actual exam. Skip that question, circle its number on your answer sheet, and move on.

When you have completed the self-test section, compare your answers to the key provided. Write down the subject and/or reference page number for each incorrect or skipped answer. Then refer to your text and study that material.

After you have studied, retake the self test. If you again have difficulty with some subjects, return to your text and repeat your review. The more often you are able to repeat this process, the better you will fare on your examination.

As you are retaking the self-tests, begin to practice timing yourself. Most examinations allow one minute per question: 60 questions, one-hour time limit; 150 questions, 2 ½-hour time limit, and so on. Timed practice sessions will actually help you to increase your test-taking speed. This will afford you extra time for the questions that require extra thought.

Learn not to allow yourself to become "bogged down" on a difficult or confusing question. You can skip it and come back. When you do skip a question, however, make sure you also skip the corresponding answer sheet entry! Although everyone will warn you about making "unnecessary stray marks or erasures," it is better to *lightly* circle the number of a skipped question than to cause all your subsequent questions to be incorrectly answered. Make sure that you erase all extra marks before submitting your sheet.

If you have co-workers or friends who will be taking the same exam, get together and do group study sessions during the week or two before the test (especially in preparation for practical examinations). Sometimes "teaching" is the best way to study.

Okay. You've done all that "good student" stuff. You've done your homework and practiced your skills, but you're still fearful and uncertain. What *more* can you do? You can relax.

Be sure to get a good night's sleep before the test. If you stay up all night studying you'll certainly do more harm than good. If you've delayed your review and can't avoid last-minute studying, you *still* should go to bed early! But then get up early and study the morning of the test, ideally over a good breakfast. If you are one of those "night shift" people who cannot mentate in the early hours of morning, you will need to arrange for a good sleep the previous afternoon and evening.

Let us pause here, and discuss the definition of a "good breakfast." Guess what? Contrary to popular EMT behavior (of all levels), a good breakfast does not consist of coffee and doughnuts. Whether or not you adopt good nutrition in your normal day-to-day living, it will be to your great advantage to do so on the morning of an event as stressful as an examination.

First, the sugar contained in the doughnuts will quickly peak, producing lethargy, while the caffeine in the coffee will provide artificial stimulation. Do you truly want to approach an exam situation *sideways*?

A breakfast high in complex carbohydrates along with some protein is the key to the sustained energy levels you'll need during a high-stress situation. Lean meats, eggs, and milk products (such as yogurt, cheeses, and low-fat milk) are good sources of protein. Carbohydrates are found in things like fresh fruits and juices, whole-grain breads, pancakes, and rice products.

A truly "good" breakfast will fuel your body, consume energy slowly and efficiently, and help you to perform at your best. An important point to remember, however; the largest shunting of blood supply to the stomach (instead of to the brain) is immediately after ingestion of food. Allow yourself a couple of hours between breakfast and test-taking. In this way, your body will be sending energy and nutrients to your brain at the time you sit for the test.

Structured review, sleep, and efficient nutrition will give you an undeniable "edge" and improve your performance in any testing situation.

Suggestions for Practical Examination Preparation and Execution

Throughout your entire EMS career you will periodically be subjected to the dreaded practical skills examination stations. They accompany all levels of EMS courses, certification exams, recertification exams, and the National Registry examination. More and more often, practical stations also accompany continuing education workshops (such as Critical Trauma Care or Pre-Hospital Trauma Life Support). Even the most veteran of EMS providers tremble in their boots when faced with the ordeal of performing in the situational exam station environment.

Why?

Skills and performance, knowledge and physical abilities are placed under the strictest scrutiny. Its unnerving to be observed and evaluated, especially when your livelihood is threatened should you fail. Even the best simulations contain components that must be recognized and remembered although you never actually see, feel, hear, or smell them. You frequently are either alone or paired with people you have never worked with before. The equipment you are given is rarely in the configuration you are accustomed to. Consequently, you may fumble around, hunting for instruments that your hands would normally find on their own. Often, when you do find the equipment, it is of a different brand, make, or model, and is unfamiliar. In addition to all the above, the evaluators themselves may appear to be "out to get you." In their effort to remain unbiased and objective, even the friendliest evaluators suddenly appear cold and perhaps hostile.

What can you do about these dilemmas?

Of course, regardless of the volume of calls you actually respond to, it is imperative that you remain skilled at operating all EMS equipment, and that you frequently refresh yourself regarding patient assessment and treatment. Periodic practice and review is essential. Volunteering your time for the testing of others is helpful in developing awareness of common performance mistakes. But the biggest improvement between past and present performances can be made by changing your approach to the situational or practical exam station itself.

When appearing for a written exam, you bring your own pencil and eraser, do you not? A similar rule applies to any practical exam station. At the very least, wear your own, old-faithful holster. This puts vital items like scissors, penlight, pens, and the like at your fingertips, just where you are accustomed to finding them. Your own stethoscope ought to be draped, bundled, or strapped about whatever it is usually draped, bundled, or strapped. Actually changing into your uniform before going through the stations is ideal. This may appear "gung-ho" to others, but these others are not grading your performance. Indeed, if you have your own emergency care kit, bring it. Your goal should be to clothe and equip yourself in a manner that makes you feel comfortable and makes your surroundings as familiar as possible.

The previous suggestions are easily applied to any practical exam station. The "assessment" or "situation" stations present a greater challenge, however. Here, the most difficult and most vital improvement you can make is in your performance style itself.

RULES FOR SITUATIONAL PRACTICAL SKILLS STATIONS

1. *Fix your eyes and your attention on the evaluator.* As you enter this station, do not preoccupy yourself with eyeing the patient or the scene to get "a head start" on the situation. Fix your eyes and your attention on the evaluator. Concentrate on the instructions and information she/he is providing.

2. *If you are offered time to examine the equipment, do it.* Look at it carefully, especially if it differs from the equipment you are accustomed to using. If possible, arrange it in a manner that is familiar to you. Do not leave it in a messy pile beside the patient.

3. *When the evaluator describes the scenario, be alert for indications of the mechanism of injury or descriptions of the scene* that cannot be simulated. If you are told that the steering wheel is bent, or the windshield fractured, or the furniture broken, *it means something.* Take time to consider the information these clues provide.

   If this type of information is not offered, *you must ask for it.* What is the condition of his apartment? Is it tidy? Messy? What does it smell like? What does the car look like? Where was the point of impact, and where was the patient sitting? Did the patient wear her/his seat belt? Is there compartmental intrusion involving the patient's space? Is the steering wheel bent/broken? Is there glass damage?

4. *As you are directed to begin, no matter what the situation, the first words you utter are "Is the scene safe?"* In real life you can see smoke on approach, smell a gas leak, hear a domestic altercation, or observe that the police have not yet arrived. For situational exams, however, the first words out of your mouth must be "Is the scene safe?"

5. *From this moment on, there is no longer any reason for you to look at the evaluator.* This is very important. Looking back and forth between the evaluator and the patient is distracting. It will interrupt your concentration and continuity. Focus your eyes and attention on the scene and the patient. Your eyes and hands should never leave the patient (except to obtain equipment). The evaluator doesn't need to see your face. She/he is listening to what you say and watching your skills performance as much as possible.

6. *Never stop talking.* Whether you are questioning the evaluator, questioning the patient, or describing your actions, you should never stop talking. Frequently, evaluators miss actions/skills performed by the testing party secondary to making notes on a skills performance sheet. Verbalize every single thing you are doing, everything you are *thinking.*

7. *Don't forget to talk to your patient.* This may sound difficult, but it can be easily incorporated with the previous suggestion. Since you should be addressing your attention to the patient but verbalizing all your thoughts and actions for the evaluator, *tell the patient what you are thinking and doing.* As often as you are able, address all your questions to the patient.

8. *If the patient doesn't have the answers, ask the evaluator, but do not remove your eye contact from the patient.* The evaluator is in the same room. She/he can hear you without your needing to look at her/him.

What follows is a written example of what a situational practical skills station should *sound like*:

EVALUATOR: You may begin.

PERFORMER: Is the scene safe?

EVALUATOR: The scene is safe.

PERFORMER: Then I am observing the scene as I approach.

Is the mechanism of injury apparent?

I can see that my patient has some blood on his left thigh. Is the blood spurting?

First, I place my hand on his head and assess his level of consciousness.

Sir? Sir? Can you hear me?

Hi. My name is Mork. I'm an Emergency Medical Technician and I'm here to help you. I need you to keep very still and not move your head.

Any pain in your neck as I run my fingers down it?

My invisible partner, Mindy, is going to hold your head to help you keep it absolutely still. She will not stop holding your head until we have you secured to a long backboard.

What's your name?

Okay, Endor, first I'd like to check your airway. I'm going to look inside and make sure it's clear. Anything loose in there, Endor?

Good. Are you having any difficulty breathing?

When I listen to his chest with this stethoscope, can I hear any unusual noises when he breathes?

Does your chest hurt at all when I compress it?

It feels even in excursion and I don't feel any crepitus or see any wounds or deformities.

My invisible partner, Mindy, will observe your airway and respiratory effort as she continues to immobilize your C-spine, and alert me to any changes while I examine you further.

I'm going to check his pulses now. Do I feel his radial pulse?

What quality and rate do I feel?

Is he sweaty?

What is his skin color?

Temperature?

Endor, I'm going to give you some oxygen to help you feel better. This is a nasal cannula and may tickle your nose a bit, but I'll run it at four liters per minute and it will help you.

Yes, an evaluator could be scoring this performance over the telephone!

A continuous narration of your thoughts and activities assists your score in a number of ways. It keeps you focused on your patient and your task, ensuring that you proceed without forgetting things. This extra degree of attention focusing also helps to calm you down, improving your physical and mental concentration. Perhaps most importantly, verbalizing everything you do and think will make it nearly impossible for the evaluator to miss what you have done. Without this technique, the evaluator may miss your sweeping check of the patient's clothing for gross bleeding because she/he was making notes on the skills performance sheet.

GROUP APPROACHES TO THE SITUATIONAL EXAM STATION

All the previous suggestions apply here as well. However, now you are working with other participants, who frequently were total strangers only moments ago. The old adage, "Too many cooks spoil the broth," applies here in quadruplicate. Few things are as debilitating and disastrous as having two, three, or four EMTs crawling all over each other, trying to treat a patient at the same time.

The secret is *organization and assignment of tasks.* Each group member must have an assigned task, with an assigned group leader in charge. As each new station is approached, the tasks must be clearly reassigned to allow each participant an opportunity to rotate through each different task performance.

Groups of two are easy. For trauma situational exam stations, one partner is Group Leader and the other is the C-spine/ Airway Monitor. The Group Leader introduces self and partner, directing partner to maintain immobilization of the C-spine continuously and to monitor for changes in airway status after the initial examination. The Group Leader examines the patient and performs all necessary treatment.

The C-spine/Airway Monitor maintains spinal immobilization and observes airway/respiratory status no matter how tempted she/he is to help with other treatment. While doing so, however, she/he may *verbally* assist whenever the Group Leader seems to have forgotten something.

For groups of two in the medical situational exam stations the C-spine/Airway Monitor becomes an "Equipment Operator." The Equipment Operator manages oxygen equipment, takes vital signs, applies the EKG monitor, positions the backboard and/or pram, and so on. The Group Leader is still responsible for the patient examination. But when an Equipment Operator is present, the Group Leader may direct application of treatments.

Groups of three responders are broken down into assignments of the Group Leader, the C-spine/Airway Monitor, and the Equipment Operator.

Groups of four responders may be broken down into assignments of the Group Leader, the C-spine Immobilizer, the Airway Monitor, and the Equipment Operator. If active airway maintenance is not required, the Airway Monitor becomes a secondary Equipment Operator. And the C-spine Immobilizer resumes observation of the airway.

If you have the misfortune of operating in a five-or-more-member team, send the fifth-or-more members to direct traffic!

The most important key to group performance, no matter how you designate the tasks, is that the assignments are clearly understood by each member.

In summary:

1. Wear your own equipment holster and stethoscope. Bring your own kit if you have one, and wear your uniform. Make the testing environment more comfortable and familiar.

2. As you first enter the station, fix your eyes and attention on the evaluator. Don't "jump the gun." Listen to the clues that the evaluator provides. Take the time to check the equipment provided. Ask for scene or situation information if it is not offered.

3. "Is the scene safe?"

4. After beginning your performance, never let your eyes or hands leave the patient.

5. Never stop talking. Talk to the patient, ask questions, and describe everything you are thinking and doing. Don't look away from the patient to ask questions of the evaluator—she/he does not need to see your face to answer you.

6. Clearly assign specific tasks to group members and take turns with task performance.

7. Do not physically deviate from your assigned task. However, you may verbally remind partners of business if they appear to have forgotten something.

8. Above all, try to enjoy yourself. Take pride in the performance level you have worked so hard to achieve, and have confidence in your abilities.

1

Test Section One

Test Section One covers the following subjects:

* Roles and Responsibilities
* EMS Terminology
* Medical Ethics
* Legal Aspects of EMS
* Extrication and Rescue
* Communications
* Ambulance Operations
* Anatomy and Physiology
* Patient Assessment
* Medical Terminology

EMT - Basic
National Standards Review Self Test

1. The EMT's primary responsibilities include
   (a) ensuring personal safety.
   (b) providing prehospital care to victims of emergencies.
   (c) transporting patients safely and expeditiously to the hospital.
   (d) All of the above.
   (e) None of the above.

2. The EMT may gather information as to what is probably wrong with the patient from the
   (a) scene.
   (b) bystanders.
   (c) patient interview.
   (d) All of the above.
   (e) None of the above.

3. An EMT may be convicted of negligence only if which of the following is proven to have occurred?
   (a) The EMT had a duty to act and care for the patient.
   (b) The EMT failed to care for the patient.
   (c) The patient was injured by the EMT's actions.
   (d) All of the above.
   (e) None of the above.

4. An EMT's best protection when involved in a lawsuit relating to a call is
   (a) a good EMS lawyer.
   (b) accurate, detailed completion of the written report.
   (c) a more experienced partner.
   (d) stating, "I cannot remember," as often as possible.
   (e) police testimony.

5. In a court of law the EMT-Basic is measured against a "standard of care." Which of the following elements is not included in this standard of care?
   (a) The community conduct of the EMT
   (b) The local legal statutes, ordinances, or case laws regarding EMS
   (c) American Heart Association CPR guidelines

(d) The Department of Transportation (DOT) national standards for emergency care

(e) The EMT-Basic textbook used in training the EMT

6. Which of the following statements regarding "actual consent" is false?

(a) To be effective, it must be informed consent.

(b) Oral consent is valid.

(c) A consent form does not eliminate the need for conversation.

(d) All of the above are false.

(e) None of the above is false.

7. You have transferred a nursing-home resident to the emergency room for evaluation of a urinary problem. As you arrive, your dispatcher notifies you of an emergency call waiting. All of the ER nurses are busy, but the clerk listens to your report and assures you that she will inform the nurse. You leave the patient in the care of the clerk. Which of the following statements regarding this situation is true?

(a) In the United States of America, this is viewed as abandonment.

(b) Only some states view this as abandonment.

(c) Emergency calls take precedence over transfers; therefore, this is not abandonment.

(d) You have completed the transfer to the ER because the patient was received by the ER clerk; therefore, this is not abandonment.

(e) None of these statements is true.

8. Which of the following statements regarding "implied consent" is false?

(a) To be effective, it must be informed consent.

(b) With any unconscious patient, the law assumes that the patient would give her/his consent.

(c) If there is a significant risk of death, the law assumes that the unconscious patient would give her/his consent.

(d) All of the above are false.

(e) None of the above is false.

9. In cases where the patient is unable to give consent but has life-threatening problems, you may provide care under the law of

    (a) implied consent.
    (b) informed consent.
    (c) actual consent.
    (d) involuntary consent.
    (e) unconscious consent.

10. In some states consent may be given by a minor if the minor is

    (a) baby-sitting other minor children.
    (b) not under the influence of alcohol or drugs.
    (c) married or pregnant.
    (d) All of the above.
    (e) None of the above.

11. Some states have "Good Samaritan Laws." These laws grant immunity from prosecution

    (a) to EMTs who operate under a physician's license.
    (b) to EMTs who have lawsuits filed against them.
    (c) to those who volunteer to help an injured person at the scene of an accident.
    (d) All of the above.
    (e) None of the above.

12. Which of the following best defines *lateral rotation*?

    (a) Standing in an upright position.
    (b) To straighten a joint.
    (c) To bend a joint.
    (d) To turn a joint or limb away from the body's midline.
    (e) To turn a joint or limb toward the body's midline.

13. Which of the following best defines *extension*?

    (a) Standing in an upright position.
    (b) To straighten a joint.
    (c) To bend a joint.
    (d) To turn a joint or limb away from the body's midline.
    (e) To turn a joint or limb toward the body's midline.

14. Which of the following best defines *medial rotation*?

    (a) Standing in an upright position.
    (b) To straighten a joint.

   (c) To bend a joint.
   (d) To turn a joint or limb away from the body's midline.
   (e) To turn a joint or limb toward the body's midline.

15. Which of the following best defines *flexion*?
   (a) Standing in an upright position.
   (b) To straighten a joint.
   (c) To bend a joint.
   (d) To turn a joint or limb away from the body's midline.
   (e) To turn a joint or limb toward the body's midline.

16. Anatomy is the study of
   (a) body structure.
   (b) body function.
   (c) body strength.
   (d) All of the above.
   (e) None of the above.

17. Physiology is the study of
   (a) body structure.
   (b) body function.
   (c) body strength.
   (d) All of the above.
   (e) None of the above.

18. *The anatomical position* refers to the human body in which position?
   (a) Standing upright with arms outstretched above the head.
   (b) Lying prone with arms along the side of the body.
   (c) Lying supine with arms along the side of the body.
   (d) All of the above.
   (e) None of the above.

19. The thumb is on the _____ side of the hand.
   (a) superior
   (b) medial
   (c) midline
   (d) inferior
   (e) lateral

20.   The umbilicus is located in the _____ of the abdomen.
   - (a) superior
   - (b) medial
   - (c) midline
   - (d) inferior
   - (e) lateral

21.   The tibia is _____ to the femur.
   - (a) superior
   - (b) medial
   - (c) midline
   - (d) inferior
   - (e) lateral

22.   The cranium is _____ to the spine.
   - (a) superior
   - (b) medial
   - (c) midline
   - (d) inferior
   - (e) lateral

23.   The great toe is on the _____ side of the foot.
   - (a) superior
   - (b) medial
   - (c) midline
   - (d) inferior
   - (e) lateral

24.   The ulna is _____ to the humerus.
   - (a) proximal
   - (b) anterior
   - (c) superior
   - (d) posterior
   - (e) distal

25.   The sternum is _____ to the thoracic spine.
   - (a) proximal
   - (b) anterior
   - (c) superior
   - (d) posterior
   - (e) distal

26. The tarsals are _____ to the metatarsals.
    (a) proximal
    (b) anterior
    (c) superior
    (d) posterior
    (e) distal

27. The cervical spine is _____ to the esophagus.
    (a) proximal
    (b) anterior
    (c) superior
    (d) posterior
    (e) distal

28. In the anatomical position, the palm of the hand is considered to be
    (a) proximal.
    (b) superior.
    (c) anterior.
    (d) inferior.
    (e) posterior.

29. A person in the supine position is lying
    (a) on her/his stomach.
    (b) on her/his side.
    (c) on the floor.
    (d) on a bed with her/his head elevated 40 degrees.
    (e) on her/his back.

30. A person in the prone position is lying
    (a) on her/his stomach.
    (b) on her/his side.
    (c) on the floor.
    (d) on a bed with her/his head elevated 40 degrees.
    (e) on her/his back.

31. A person in the lateral recumbent position is lying
    (a) on her/his stomach.
    (b) on her/his side.
    (c) on the floor.
    (d) on a bed with her/his head elevated 40 degrees.
    (e) on her/his back.

32.   In the medical sense, *abduction* refers to
   (a) movement toward the body.
   (b) movement toward the head.
   (c) movement away from the body.
   (d) movement toward the feet.
   (e) movement toward the back.

33.   *Adduction* refers to
   (a) movement toward the body.
   (b) movement toward the head.
   (c) movement away from the body.
   (d) movement toward the feet.
   (e) movement toward the back.

34.   The skull consists of
   (a) the cranium (which contains the brain) only.
   (b) the cranium (which contains the brain) and the face.
   (c) the cranium (which contains the brain), the face, and the first vertebra of the spine.
   (d) the cranium (which contains the brain), the face, and the first two vertebrae of the spine.
   (e) None of the above.

35.   Which of the following statements regarding the spinal column is false?
   (a) The spinal column encloses the spinal cord.
   (b) The spinal cord connects with the brain through an opening at the base of the skull.
   (c) The spinal column consists of 33 bones known as vertebrae.
   (d) The spine is divided into five sections.
   (e) The coccyx does not enclose any portion of the spinal cord, and therefore is part of the pelvic girdle.

36.   The sacrum is the section of the spine located
   (a) in the upper back, having ribs attached to it.
   (b) immediately inferior to the lower back.
   (c) at the most superior area of the spine.
   (d) in the neck.
   (e) at the most inferior area of the spine.

37.   The thoracic section of the spine is located
   (a) in the upper back, having ribs attached to it.
   (b) immediately inferior to the lower back.

(c) in the lower back and does not have attached ribs.
(d) in the neck.
(e) at the most inferior area of the spine.

38. The cervical section of the spine is located
    (a) in the upper back, having ribs attached to it.
    (b) immediately inferior to the lower back.
    (c) in the lower back and does not have attached ribs.
    (d) in the neck.
    (e) at the most inferior area of the spine.

39. The coccyx is the section of the spine located
    (a) in the upper back, having ribs attached to it.
    (b) immediately inferior to the lower back.
    (c) in the lower back and does not have attached ribs.
    (d) in the neck.
    (e) at the most inferior area of the spine.

40. The lumbar section of the spine is located
    (a) in the upper back, having ribs attached to it.
    (b) immediately inferior to the lower back.
    (c) in the lower back and does not have attached ribs.
    (d) in the neck.
    (e) at the most inferior area of the spine.

41. The abdominal cavity and thoracic cavity are separated by the
    (a) duodenum.
    (b) xiphoid process.
    (c) lower rib margin.
    (d) cerebellum.
    (e) diaphragm.

42. If a patient sustained a blunt injury to the right upper quadrant of the abdomen, which organ would you be primarily concerned about?
    (a) The heart.
    (b) The intestines.
    (c) The liver.
    (d) The spleen.
    (e) The appendix.

43. If a patient sustained a penetrating injury to the left lower quadrant of the abdomen, which organ would you be primarily concerned about?

    (a) The heart.
    (b) The intestines.
    (c) The liver.
    (d) The spleen.
    (e) The appendix.

44. If a patient sustained a blunt injury to the left upper quadrant of the abdomen, which organ would you be primarily concerned about?

    (a) The heart.
    (b) The intestines.
    (c) The liver.
    (d) The spleen.
    (e) The appendix.

45. If a patient complained of severe pain in the right lower quadrant of the abdomen, which organ would you be primarily concerned about?

    (a) The heart.
    (b) The intestines.
    (c) The liver.
    (d) The spleen.
    (e) The appendix.

46. The carotid pulse is located in the patient's

    (a) wrist.
    (b) groin.
    (c) upper arm.
    (d) neck.
    (e) foot.

47. The radial pulse is located in the patient's

    (a) wrist.
    (b) groin.
    (c) upper arm.
    (d) neck.
    (e) foot.

48. The brachial pulse is located in the patient's

    (a) wrist.
    (b) groin.

       (c) upper arm.

       (d) neck.

       (e) foot.

49. The femoral pulse is located in the patient's
- (a) wrist.
- (b) groin.
- (c) upper arm.
- (d) neck.
- (e) foot.

50. The pedal pulse is located in the patient's
- (a) wrist.
- (b) groin.
- (c) upper arm.
- (d) neck.
- (e) foot.

51. Auscultation refers to the process of
- (a) listening to areas of the body with a stethoscope.
- (b) systematically gathering information from the patient.
- (c) touching and feeling the patient to detect injuries or pain.
- (d) watching the patient closely for changes in level of consciousness.
- (e) tapping on the chest or abdomen.

52. Palpation refers to the process of
- (a) listening to areas of the body with a stethoscope.
- (b) systematically gathering information from the patient.
- (c) touching and feeling the patient to detect injuries or pain.
- (d) watching the patient closely for changes in level of consciousness.
- (e) tapping on the chest or abdomen.

53. A primary survey requires that the EMT assess
- (a) respiratory effort.
- (b) level of consciousness.
- (c) circulatory status.
- (d) All of the above.
- (e) None of the above.

54. When opening the airway of a patient who you suspect may have spine injuries, the most appropriate method is the

    (a) head-tilt, chin-lift maneuver.
    (b) Jaw-thrust maneuver.
    (c) head-tilt, neck-lift maneuver.
    (d) Any of the above.
    (e) None of the above.

55. When assessing a pulse, the EMT should note

    (a) the rate, strength, and regularity.
    (b) the pulse pressure.
    (c) the temperature and color.
    (d) All of the above.
    (e) None of the above.

56. During the primary survey, an example of bleeding that must be controlled is

    (a) a nosebleed.
    (b) a venous bleed.
    (c) an arterial bleed.
    (d) All of the above.
    (e) None of the above.

57. In the secondary survey, the EMT is concerned with

    (a) checking for and controlling life-threatening problems.
    (b) checking for and stabilizing injuries not threatening to life.
    (c) calling in the radio report.
    (d) All of the above.
    (e) None of the above.

58. The Glasgow Coma Scale is a scoring system that assesses

    (a) motor, verbal, and eye-opening responses.
    (b) orientation to person, place, and time.
    (c) blood pressure, capillary refill, respiratory rate.
    (d) pupillary response, neck movement, and mentation.
    (e) respiratory rate and excursion.

59. In the phrase, "signs and symptoms," a sign is

    (a) something a bystander saw the patient do.
    (b) something the patient refuses to explain.
    (c) something the rescuer notices about the scene.
    (d) something the patient tells about himself.
    (e) something the rescuer sees, hears, feels, or smells.

60.   In the phrase, "signs and symptoms," a symptom is
      (a) something a bystander saw the patient do.
      (b) something the patient refuses to explain.
      (c) something the rescuer notices about the scene.
      (d) something the patient tells about himself.
      (e) something the rescuer sees, hears, feels, or smells.

61.   The color of cyanosis is described as being
      (a) red.
      (b) white.
      (c) normal.
      (d) blue.
      (e) yellow.

62.   The color of jaundice is described as being
      (a) red.
      (b) white.
      (c) normal.
      (d) blue.
      (e) yellow.

63.   A patient's pale skin color suggests the possibility of
      (a) liver disease.
      (b) shock.
      (c) infectious disease.
      (d) All of the above.
      (e) None of the above.

64.   A patient's jaundiced skin color suggests the possibility of
      (a) liver disease.
      (b) shock.
      (c) high blood pressure.
      (d) All of the above.
      (e) None of the above.

65.   A patient's red, "flushed" skin color suggests the possibility of
      (a) high blood pressure.
      (b) infectious disease.
      (c) alcohol abuse.
      (d) All of the above.
      (e) None of the above.

66.   The normal resting pulse rate for adults is
   (a) 40 to 60 beats per minute.
   (b) 60 to 80 beats per minute.
   (c) 80 to 100 beats per minute.
   (d) All of the above.
   (e) None of the above.

67.   The normal resting pulse rate for children is
   (a) 40 to 60 beats per minute.
   (b) 60 to 80 beats per minute.
   (c) 80 to 100 beats per minute.
   (d) All of the above.
   (e) None of the above.

68.   The normal respiratory rate for an adult is
   (a) between 10 and 12 breaths per minute.
   (b) between 12 and 20 breaths per minute.
   (c) between 20 and 28 breaths per minute.
   (d) All of the above.
   (e) None of the above.

69.   The normal respiratory rate for an infant is
   (a) between 10 and 12 breaths per minute.
   (b) between 12 and 20 breaths per minute.
   (c) between 20 and 28 breaths per minute.
   (d) All of the above.
   (e) None of the above.

70.   The normal respiratory rate for a child is
   (a) between 10 and 12 breaths per minute.
   (b) between 12 and 20 breaths per minute.
   (c) between 20 and 28 breaths per minute.
   (d) All of the above.
   (e) None of the above.

71.   The diastolic blood pressure represents
   (a) the pressure that the circulating blood exerts against the walls of the arteries during the relaxation of the heart.
   (b) the pressure that the circulating blood exerts against the walls of the veins during contraction of the heart.
   (c) the pressure that the circulating blood exerts against the walls of the veins during relaxation of the heart.

(d) the pressure that the circulating blood exerts against the walls of the arteries during contraction of the heart.
(e) the amount of time it takes the blood to circulate within the body.

72. The systolic blood pressure represents
(a) the pressure that the circulating blood exerts against the walls of the arteries during the relaxation of the heart.
(b) the pressure that the circulating blood exerts against the walls of the veins during contraction of the heart.
(c) the pressure that the circulating blood exerts against the walls of the veins during relaxation of the heart.
(d) the pressure that the circulating blood exerts against the walls of the arteries during contraction of the heart.
(e) the amount of time it takes the blood to circulate within the body.

73. When auscultating a blood pressure, the point at which you first hear the pulse is the
(a) venous blood pressure.
(b) arterial blood pressure.
(c) diastolic blood pressure.
(d) palpated blood pressure.
(e) systolic blood pressure.

74. When auscultating a blood pressure, the point at which you last hear the pulse is the
(a) venous blood pressure.
(b) arterial blood pressure.
(c) diastolic blood pressure.
(d) palpated blood pressure.
(e) systolic blood pressure.

75. The blood pressure that is measured without a stethoscope is called a
(a) venous blood pressure.
(b) arterial blood pressure.
(c) diastolic blood pressure.
(d) palpated blood pressure.
(e) systolic blood pressure.

76.   When a blood pressure is measured without a stethoscope,
      the point at which you first feel the pulse is the
      (a) venous blood pressure.
      (b) arterial blood pressure.
      (c) diastolic blood pressure.
      (d) palpated blood pressure.
      (e) systolic blood pressure.

77.   When a blood pressure is measured without a stethoscope,
      you cannot obtain the
      (a) venous blood pressure.
      (b) arterial blood pressure.
      (c) diastolic blood pressure.
      (d) palpated blood pressure.
      (e) systolic blood pressure.

78.   In a multiple-casualty situation, which of the following
      patients should receive the highest priority of care?
      (a) A 30-year-old male with a fractured right arm.
      (b) A 3-year-old male with a fractured right arm.
      (c) A 30-year-old male with a head injury and altered
          mentation.
      (d) A 20-year-old female who has agonal respirations with
          massive facial trauma, a crushing chest injury, and an
          eviscerated abdomen.
      (e) A 30-year-old female with second-degree thermal burns
          about both lower legs.

79.   In a multiple-casualty situation, which of the following
      patients should receive the second highest priority of care?
      (a) A 30-year-old male with a fractured right arm.
      (b) A 3-year-old male with a fractured right arm.
      (c) A 30-year-old male with a head injury and altered
          mentation.
      (d) A 20-year-old female who has agonal respirations with
          massive facial trauma, a crushing chest injury, and an
          eviscerated abdomen.
      (e) A 30-year-old female with second-degree thermal burns
          about both lower legs.

80.   In a multiple-casualty situation, which of the following
      patients should receive the lowest priority of care?
      (a) A 30-year-old male with a fractured right arm.
      (b) A 3-year-old male with a fractured right arm.

    (c) A 30-year-old male with a head injury and altered mentation.

    (d) A 20-year-old female who has agonal respirations with massive facial trauma, a crushing chest injury, and an eviscerated abdomen.

    (e) A 30-year-old female with second-degree thermal burns about both lower legs.

81. *Triage* is defined as

    (a) counting the number of casualties and separating them into equal groups for rapid care.

    (b) a French term meaning "the officer who counts."

    (c) sorting multiple casualties into priorities for emergency care.

    (d) All of the above.

    (e) None of the above.

82. Which of the following statements regarding ambulance operation is false?

    (a) All states require a full stop prior to entering an intersection against a red light.

    (b) Use of lights and sirens does not guarantee that opposing traffic will yield to the ambulance.

    (c) When an ambulance is not on an emergency call, all laws applicable to private vehicle operation also apply to ambulance operation.

    (d) All of the above are false.

    (e) None of the above is false.

83. If the ambulance begins to hydroplane on a wet road

    (a) quickly apply the brakes.

    (b) turn the wheel from side to side to break through.

    (c) slowly accelerate until you are clear.

    (d) slowly decelerate by releasing the accelerator.

    (e) maintain present speed and steer for the nearest curb.

84. Of the following situations/conditions, which is the most hazardous to vehicle operations?

    (a) Driving in rain.

    (b) Driving in snow or sleet.

    (c) Driving at dawn or dusk.

    (d) Driving in fog or mist.

    (e) Driving on highways.

85.   Which of the following statements regarding police escort for
an emergency ambulance response is false?

  (a) Police escort always reduces the possibility of having an
accident en route to a call.

  (b) It is important to follow the police car as closely as
possible so that a private vehicle cannot move between
the police car and the ambulance.

  (c) All EMS systems recommend police escort when
available.

  (d) All of the above are false.

  (e) None of the above is false.

86.   At the scene of a hazardous-material spill, the ambulance
should be parked

  (a) upwind and 2000 ft from the site of the accident.

  (b) downwind and 100 ft from the site of the accident.

  (c) downwind and 500 ft from the site of the accident.

  (d) upwind and 50 ft from the site of the accident.

  (e) downwind and 2000 ft from the site of the accident.

87.   Which of the following statements regarding EMT safety in
lifting and moving patients is false?

  (a) Do not try to handle too heavy a load. When in doubt,
call for help.

  (b) Avoid twisting when lifting, lowering, or pulling.

  (c) When lifting a heavy patient, keep your back straight
and rely on shoulder and leg muscles.

  (d) When pulling a heavy patient, keep your back straight
and pull, using the arms and shoulders.

  (e) Keep in mind that it is easier to lower a heavy patient
than to lift a heavy patient.

88.   The major danger in moving a trauma patient quickly is the
possibility of

  (a) causing a long bone fracture to move.

  (b) causing increased pain.

  (c) causing spine injury.

  (d) separating fractured bone ends.

  (e) causing loss of limb.

89.   Which of the following statements regarding life-threatening
emergency moves of a patient is true?

  (a) Every effort should be made to pull the patient in the
direction of the long axis of the body.

  (b) It is impossible to remove a patient from a vehicle

quickly and, at the same time, provide protection for the spine.

(c) A patient on the floor may be dragged away from the scene by grasping the clothing in the neck and shoulder area.

(d) All of the above are true.

(e) None of the above is true.

90. Which of the following statements regarding written documentation of an emergency call is false?

(a) Written reports provide for continuity of care.

(b) Written reports furnish a source of information for evaluating quality of care.

(c) Written reports furnish legal evidence in a court of law.

(d) All of the above are false.

(e) None of the above is false.

91. The medical term for a collection of blood under the skin after blunt trauma is

(a) hemorrhage.

(b) hematomegaly.

(c) hematuria.

(d) hematoma.

(e) hemourine.

92. The medical term for external bleeding is

(a) hemorrhage.

(b) hematomegaly.

(c) hematuria.

(d) hematoma.

(e) hemourine.

93. The medical term for blood in the urine is

(a) hemorrhage.

(b) hematomegaly.

(c) hematuria.

(d) hematoma.

(e) hemourine.

94. The medical term for internal bleeding is

(a) hemorrhage.

(b) hematomegaly.

(c) hematuria.

(d) hematoma.

(e) hemourine.

95.   The medical term for vomiting blood is
  (a) vomitemia.
  (b) hematemesis.
  (c) regurgitemia.
  (d) hemasputum.
  (e) hemoptysis.

96.   The medical term for coughing up blood is
  (a) vomitemia.
  (b) hematemesis.
  (c) regurgitemia.
  (d) hemasputum.
  (e) hemoptysis.

97.   The medical term for a patient's neck being greatly manipulated backwards is
  (a) hyperflexion.
  (b) hypoflexion.
  (c) hyperextension.
  (d) hypoextension.
  (e) retrogradextension.

98.   The medical term for a patient's neck being greatly manipulated forward is
  (a) hyperflexion.
  (b) hypoflexion.
  (c) hyperextension.
  (d) hypoextension.
  (e) antegradextension.

99.   The medical term for an abnormally increased body temperature is
  (a) sweats.
  (b) hypertemperature.
  (c) hypotemperature.
  (d) hyperthermia.
  (e) hypothermia.

100. The medical term for an abnormally decreased body temperature is
  (a) chills.
  (b) hypertemperature.
  (c) hypotemperature.
  (d) hyperthermia.
  (e) hypothermia.

101. The medical term for a faster rate of breathing, with a greater depth of respiration is
  (a) hyperventilation.
  (b) hypoventilation.
  (c) hypnoventilation.
  (d) hyperoxygenation.
  (e) tachyventilation.

102. The medical term for difficulty in breathing is
  (a) hypopnea.
  (b) diffpnea.
  (c) dyspnea.
  (d) tachypnea.
  (e) hyperpnea.

103. The medical term for a rapid respiratory rate is
  (a) hypopnea.
  (b) diffpnea.
  (c) dyspnea.
  (d) tachypnea.
  (e) hyperpnea.

104. The medical term for excessively deep respirations is
  (a) hypopnea.
  (b) diffpnea.
  (c) dyspnea.
  (d) tachypnea.
  (e) hyperpnea.

105. The medical term for the act of breathing in is
  (a) inspiration/inhalation.
  (b) expiration/exhalation.
  (c) respiration/rehalation.
  (d) anterespiration/antehalation.
  (e) postrespiration/postinhalation.

106. The medical term for the act of breathing out is
  (a) inspiration/inhalation.
  (b) expiration/exhalation.
  (c) respiration/rehalation.
  (d) anterespiration/antehalation.
  (e) postrespiration/postinhalation.

107. A medical suffix meaning "surgical removal of" is

   (a) -itis.
   (b) -ictus.
   (c) -ectomy.
   (d) -ectus.
   (e) -ictal.

108. A medical suffix meaning "inflammation of" is

   (a) -itis.
   (b) -ictus.
   (c) -ectomy.
   (d) -ectus.
   (e) -ictal.

109. The medical term for an open wound with uneven, jagged edges is

   (a) cut.
   (b) incision.
   (c) cutaneous.
   (d) stoma.
   (e) laceration.

110. The medical term for an open wound with even, smooth edges is

   (a) cut.
   (b) incision.
   (c) cutaneous.
   (d) stoma.
   (e) laceration.

111. The medical term for a bruise is

   (a) hematoma.
   (b) contusion.
   (c) hemaderma.
   (d) eurythemia.
   (e) abrasion.

112. The medical term for a simple scraping injury is

   (a) hematoma.
   (b) contusion.
   (c) hemaderma.
   (d) eurythemia.
   (e) abrasion.

113. The medical term for a nosebleed is
- (a) epistaxis.
- (b) episiotomy.
- (c) epidural.
- (d) rhinorhea.
- (e) rhinohemia.

114. The medical term for regurgitated matter is
- (a) regurgitus.
- (b) vomit.
- (c) puke.
- (d) emesis.
- (e) gastritis.

115. The medical term for "passing out" but quickly regaining consciousness is
- (a) fainting spell.
- (b) feigned faint.
- (c) stuporous.
- (d) syncope.
- (e) sluggish.

116. The medical term for the feeling of impending regurgitation is
- (a) noxious.
- (b) sick.
- (c) nausea.
- (d) vomitus.
- (e) emesis.

117. The medical term for the complaint "The room is spinning!" is
- (a) vitaligo.
- (b) dizzy.
- (c) light-headedness.
- (d) vertigo.
- (e) vestigal.

118. The medical term for "running a temperature" is
- (a) feverish.
- (b) febrile.
- (c) hypothermia.
- (d) eurythemia.
- (e) hypertemperature.

119. The medical prefix that means "without" or "lack of" is
    (a) anti-.
    (b) ecto-.
    (c) iso-.
    (d) a-.
    (e) contra-.

120. The medical term for a patient's complaint or condition that is new, or of sudden onset, or especially severe is
    (a) chronic.
    (b) atypical.
    (c) acute.
    (d) obscure.
    (e) typical.

121. The medical term for a patient's complaint or condition that has persisted over a long period of time is
    (a) chronic.
    (b) atypical.
    (c) acute.
    (d) obscure.
    (e) typical.

122. The medical term for the temporary or permanent loss of voluntary movement is
    (a) hemiparaplegia.
    (b) paraplegia.
    (c) paralysis.
    (d) hemiplegia.
    (e) quadriplegia.

123. The medical term for the loss of voluntary movement on one side of the body is
    (a) hemiparaplegia.
    (b) paraplegia.
    (c) paralysis.
    (d) hemiplegia.
    (e) quadriplegia.

124. The medical term for the loss of voluntary movement in the lower portion of the body and both legs is
    (a) hemiparaplegia.
    (b) paraplegia.

(c) paralysis.
(d) hemiplegia.
(e) quadriplegia.

125. The medical term for the loss of voluntary movement in all four extremities is
   (a) hemiparaplegia.
   (b) paraplegia.
   (c) paralysis.
   (d) hemiplegia.
   (e) quadriplegia.

126. The medical term for having high blood pressure is
   (a) hypertensive.
   (b) hypotensive.
   (c) normotensive.
   (d) hyperpressured.
   (e) hypopressured.

127. The medical term for having low blood pressure is
   (a) hypertensive.
   (b) hypotensive.
   (c) normotensive.
   (d) hyperpressured.
   (e) hypopressured.

128. When pain from an illness or injury is felt in an area other than its actual location, it is called
   (a) radiation of pain.
   (b) accessory pain.
   (c) referred pain.
   (d) locomotion of pain.
   (e) drifting pain.

129. The term for the spreading of pain from an area of illness or injury into another area is
   (a) radiation of pain.
   (b) accessory pain.
   (c) referred pain.
   (d) locomotion of pain.
   (e) drifting pain.

130. The medical term for a pulse rate that is faster than normal is

    (a) tachypnea.
    (b) bradycardia.
    (c) cardiomegaly.
    (d) tachycardia.
    (e) bradychypnea.

131. The medical term for a pulse rate that is slower than normal is

    (a) tachypnea.
    (b) bradycardia.
    (c) cardiomegaly.
    (d) tachycardia.
    (e) bradychypnea.

132. If a condition or injury involves both sides of a structure, it can be described as being

    (a) trilateral.
    (b) bilateral.
    (c) unilateral.
    (d) bimedial.
    (e) unimedial.

133. If a condition or injury involves only one side of a structure, it can be described as being

    (a) trilateral.
    (b) bilateral.
    (c) unilateral.
    (d) bimedial.
    (e) unimedial.

134. When foreign liquid or solid material has been inhaled into the lungs, it is called

    (a) inspiration.
    (b) respiration.
    (c) sucking chest.
    (d) alienation.
    (e) aspiration.

135. The medical term for the absence of breathing is

    (a) anoxia.
    (b) hyperpnea.
    (c) apnea.

(d) hypoxemia.
(e) hypoxia.

136. The medical term for an inadequate supply of oxygen to the tissues of the body is
   (a) anoxia.
   (b) hyperpnea.
   (c) apnea.
   (d) hypoxemia.
   (e) hypoxia.

137. The medical term for an injury that has an entrance wound only is
   (a) stabbing wound.
   (b) obstructed wound.
   (c) perforating wound.
   (d) penetrating wound.
   (e) proximal wound.

138. The medical term for an injury that has an exit and an entrance wound is
   (a) stabbing wound.
   (b) obstructed wound.
   (c) perforating wound.
   (d) penetrating wound.
   (e) proximal wound.

139. The medical term for the supply of oxygenated blood to body parts, organs, and tissues is
   (a) profusion.
   (b) perfusion.
   (c) percussion.
   (d) procusion.
   (e) percusion.

The answer key for Test Section One is on page 213.

2

Test Section Two

Test Section Two covers the following
subjects and their treatment:

* Airway Mechanics and Obstruction
* Airway Adjuncts and Oxygen Delivery Systems
* Respiratory Arrest and Resuscitation
* Circulation
* Cardiac Arrest and CPR
* Poisons/Bites/Stings
* Heart Attack
* Stroke
* Dyspnea
* Medical Terminology

EMT - Basic
National Standards Review Self Test

1.   A gas that is a by-product of various metabolic processes within the body is called

     (a) oxygen.
     (b) carbon monoxide.
     (c) carbon dioxide.
     (d) hemoglobin.
     (e) nitrous oxide.

2.   In the lungs, oxygen is exchanged moving from the

     (a) alveoli to the capillaries.
     (b) capillaries to the body cells.
     (c) alveoli to the body cells.
     (d) capillaries to the alveoli.
     (e) body cells to the capillaries.

3.   In the body, oxygen is exchanged moving from the

     (a) alveoli to the capillaries.
     (b) capillaries to the body cells.
     (c) alveoli to the body cells.
     (d) capillaries to the alveoli.
     (e) body cells to the capillaries.

4.   In the lungs, carbon dioxide is exchanged moving from the

     (a) alveoli to the capillaries.
     (b) capillaries to the body cells.
     (c) alveoli to the body cells.
     (d) capillaries to the alveoli.
     (e) body cells to the capillaries.

5.   In the body, carbon dioxide is exchanged moving from the

     (a) alveoli to the capillaries.
     (b) capillaries to the body cells.
     (c) alveoli to the body cells.
     (d) capillaries to the alveoli.
     (e) body cells to the capillaries.

6.   Biological death begins

     (a) immediately after cessation of breathing and pulse.
     (b) within 3 to 5 minutes after cessation of breathing and pulse.

(c) within 4 to 6 minutes after cessation of breathing and pulse.

(d) 10 or more minutes after cessation of breathing and pulse.

(e) 15 or more minutes after cessation of breathing and pulse.

7. Clinical death begins

(a) immediately after cessation of breathing and pulse.

(b) within 3 to 5 minutes after cessation of breathing and pulse.

(c) within 4 to 6 minutes after cessation of breathing and pulse.

(d) 10 or more minutes after cessation of breathing and pulse.

(e) 15 or more minutes after cessation of breathing and pulse.

8. Brain damage begins

(a) immediately after cessation of breathing and pulse.

(b) within 3 to 5 minutes after cessation of breathing and pulse.

(c) within 4 to 6 minutes after cessation of breathing and pulse.

(d) 10 or more minutes after cessation of breathing and pulse.

(e) 15 or more minutes after cessation of breathing and pulse.

9. The slippery tissue covering the lungs and lining the interior chest cavity is called

(a) the cilia.

(b) the diaphragm.

(c) the alveoli.

(d) the dermis.

(e) the pleura.

10. The muscle that separates the thoracic cavity from the abdominal cavity is called

(a) the cilia.

(b) the diaphragm.

(c) the alveoli.

(d) the dermis.

(e) the pleura.

11.   In the lungs, the bronchi branch into smaller parts until
       they finally end in tiny air sacs called
            (a) the cilia.
            (b) the diaphragm.
            (c) the alveoli.
            (d) the dermis.
            (e) the pleura.

12.   Air entering the nose or mouth (or food entering the mouth)
       first passes through the
            (a) larynx.
            (b) epiglottis.
            (c) pharynx.
            (d) trachea.
            (e) bronchi.

13.   The main tube leading to the lungs branches into two
       smaller tubes called the right and left
            (a) larynx.
            (b) epiglottis.
            (c) pharynx.
            (d) trachea.
            (e) bronchi.

14.   The main tube leading to the lungs is called the
            (a) larynx.
            (b) epiglottis.
            (c) pharynx.
            (d) trachea.
            (e) bronchi.

15.   The structure that guards the tube to the lungs by closing
       whenever food or liquids are present is called the
            (a) larynx.
            (b) epiglottis.
            (c) pharynx.
            (d) trachea.
            (e) bronchi.

16.   The structure that contains the vocal cords is the
            (a) larynx.
            (b) epiglottis.

(c) pharynx.

(d) trachea.

(e) bronchi.

17. The primary airway of the respiratory system is the

   (a) larynx.

   (b) mouth.

   (c) pharynx.

   (d) nose.

   (e) trachea.

18. The secondary airway of the respiratory system is the

   (a) larynx.

   (b) mouth.

   (c) pharynx.

   (d) nose.

   (e) trachea.

19. When the diaphragm and rib muscles contract

   (a) the larynx opens and air rushes in.

   (b) the chest cavity becomes smaller and air is forced out.

   (c) the larynx opens and air rushes out.

   (d) the chest cavity enlarges and the lungs fill with air.

   (e) None of the above.

20. When the diaphragm and rib muscles relax

   (a) the larynx opens and air rushes in.

   (b) the chest cavity becomes smaller and air is forced out.

   (c) the larynx opens and air rushes out.

   (d) the chest cavity enlarges and the lungs fill with air.

   (e) None of the above.

21. The linings of the lung and chest cavity have a small amount of fluid between them, no air, and no openings to allow air in. This feature

   (a) creates a negative pressure so that the lungs will deflate with exhalation.

   (b) protects the lungs from infection.

   (c) produces a suction that allows the lungs to expand when the chest does.

   (d) All of the above.

   (e) None of the above.

22. Breathing is automatically controlled by the
   (a) brain.
   (b) diaphragm.
   (c) patient.
   (d) blood.
   (e) lungs.

23. If the respiratory center of a normal, healthy body notices a blood level of carbon dioxide that is too high, it causes the body to
   (a) breathe faster and deeper to replace the carbon dioxide with oxygen.
   (b) breathe slower and deeper to accumulate more oxygen.
   (c) breathe slower and more shallowly to "blow off" excess carbon dioxide.
   (d) continue breathing normally.
   (e) stop breathing.

24. If the respiratory center of a normal, healthy body notices a blood level of oxygen that is too low, it causes the body to
   (a) breathe faster and deeper to replace the carbon dioxide with oxygen.
   (b) breathe slower and deeper to accumulate more oxygen.
   (c) breathe slower and more shallowly to "blow off" excess carbon dioxide.
   (d) continue breathing normally.
   (e) stop breathing.

25. Breathing is considered to be adequate when
   (a) the chest and abdomen rise and fall as air is breathed in and out.
   (b) air can be quietly heard coming in and out of the nose and/or mouth.
   (c) air can be felt coming in and out of the nose and/or mouth.
   (d) All of the above.
   (e) None of the above.

26. The normal respiratory rate for an adult at rest is
   (a) 2 to 10 breaths per minute.
   (b) 10 to 25 breaths per minute.
   (c) 12 to 20 breaths per minute.
   (d) 14 to 16 breaths per minute.
   (e) 14 to 24 breaths per minute.

27. *Cyanosis* is defined as
    (a) the absence of respiratory effort.
    (b) the absence of oxygen in the blood.
    (c) pale nail beds, palms, and skin.
    (d) a grayish-blue discoloration of the skin.
    (e) a lack of oxygen in the lungs.

28. A patient who is in cardiac arrest
    (a) is not breathing but may still have a pulse.
    (b) is adequately breathing but requires chest compressions to create a pulse.
    (c) is not breathing and does not have a pulse.
    (d) Any of the above.
    (e) None of the above.

29. A patient who is in respiratory arrest
    (a) is not breathing but may still have a pulse.
    (b) is adequately breathing but requires chest compressions to create a pulse.
    (c) is not breathing and does not have a pulse.
    (d) Any of the above.
    (e) None of the above.

30. A patient who requires pulmonary resuscitation only
    (a) is not breathing but may still have a pulse.
    (b) is adequately breathing but requires chest compressions to create a pulse.
    (c) is not breathing and does not have a pulse.
    (d) Any of the above.
    (e) None of the above.

31. A patient who is in cardiopulmonary arrest
    (a) is not breathing but may still have a pulse.
    (b) is adequately breathing but requires chest compressions to create a pulse.
    (c) is not breathing and does not have a pulse.
    (d) Any of the above.
    (e) None of the above.

32.   As you approach a supine patient you notice an absence of chest movement, but the abdomen appears to quiver or spasm. This indicates that

   (a) the patient is hyperventilating and should be made to breathe into a bag.
   (b) the patient's breathing is inadequate.
   (c) the patient's abdominal muscles are trying to assist respirations.
   (d) the patient is having a localized seizure.
   (e) the patient is trying not to laugh.

33.   Uneven or very shallow chest movement indicates that

   (a) the patient is hyperventilating and should be made to breathe into a bag.
   (b) the patient's breathing is inadequate.
   (c) the patient's abdominal muscles are trying to assist respirations.
   (d) the patient is having a localized seizure.
   (e) the patient is trying not to laugh.

34.   You notice that your patient is breathing very deeply and very rapidly. This indicates

   (a) the patient is hyperventilating and should be made to breathe into a bag.
   (b) the patient's breathing is inadequate.
   (c) the patient's abdominal muscles are trying to assist respirations.
   (d) the patient is having a localized seizure.
   (e) the patient is trying not to laugh.

35.   The most frequent cause of airway obstruction is

   (a) large pieces of unchewed meat (especially steak or hot dogs).
   (b) alcohol ingestion while eating.
   (c) food ingestion during activity.
   (d) mucous plugs.
   (e) the tongue.

36.   Lifting the lower jaw with the fingers of one hand while pressing your other hand on the patient's forehead to tilt the head back is called

   (a) The head-tilt neck-lift maneuver.
   (b) The head-tilt chin-lift maneuver.
   (c) The modified jaw thrust maneuver.

    (d) Both answers (a) and (b).

    (e) Answers (a), (b), and (c).

37. Which of the following maneuvers is acceptable for the management of the unconscious, nontraumatic patient?

    (a) The head-tilt neck-lift maneuver.

    (b) The head-tilt chin-lift maneuver.

    (c) The modified jaw thrust maneuver.

    (d) Both answers (a) and (b).

    (e) Answers (a), (b), and (c).

38. Which of the following maneuvers is acceptable for the management of the unconscious trauma patient?

    (a) The head-tilt neck-lift maneuver.

    (b) The head-tilt chin-lift maneuver.

    (c) The modified jaw thrust maneuver.

    (d) Both answers (a) and (b).

    (e) Answers (a), (b), and (c).

39. Which of the following maneuvers is preferred by the American Heart Association for the management of the unconscious, nontraumatic patient?

    (a) The head-tilt neck-lift maneuver.

    (b) The head-tilt chin-lift maneuver.

    (c) The modified jaw thrust maneuver.

    (d) Both answers (a) and (b).

    (e) Answers (a), (b), and (c).

40. After correctly opening the airway, if the patient does not start breathing spontaneously, the EMT should

    (a) assess the level of consciousness.

    (b) perform 6 to 10 back blows.

    (c) provide pain stimulus to trigger respiratory effort.

    (d) check for a pulse.

    (e) immediately begin artificial respiration.

41. The atmosphere (at sea level) contains approximately _____ oxygen.

    (a) 45 percent.

    (b) 29 percent

    (c) 12 percent

    (d) 16 percent

    (e) 21 percent

42. The oxygen content of an exhaled breath is approximately
  (a) 45 percent.
  (b) 29 percent.
  (c) 12 percent.
  (d) 16 percent.
  (e) 21 percent.

43. Place the following in order of correct performance sequence.
  1. Check the pulse.
  2. Call for help.
  3. Properly position the patient and open the airway.
  4. Establish unresponsiveness.
  5. Look, listen, and feel for breathing.
  6. If breathing is absent, ventilate the patient.

  (a) 4, 2, 3, 6, 5, 1.
  (b) 1, 2, 4, 3, 6, 5.
  (c) 2, 1, 4, 3, 6, 5.
  (d) 4, 1, 3, 6, 5, 2.
  (e) 1, 4, 3, 5, 6, 2.

44. The amount of time required to determine breathlessness is
  (a) the time it takes to say, "capillary refill."
  (b) 1 to 3 seconds.
  (c) 3 to 5 seconds.
  (d) the amount of time you can comfortably hold your own breath.
  (e) 5 to 10 seconds.

45. How many breaths do you initially deliver to the patient in respiratory arrest?
  (a) One long, slow breath.
  (b) Four quick breaths (without allowing passive exhalation between them, in order to achieve a "stair-step" effect and fully reinflate the patient's collapsed lungs).
  (c) Three quick breaths (without allowing passive exhalation between them, in order to achieve a "stair-step" effect and fully reinflate the patient's collapsed lungs).
  (d) Two quick breaths (without allowing passive exhalation between them, in order to achieve a "stair-step" effect and fully reinflate the patient's collapsed lungs).
  (e) Two deep breaths, lasting 1 to 1.5 seconds (allowing passive exhalation between them).

46. You know that your ventilations are inadequate when
   (a) the chest is seen to rise and fall with each breath.
   (b) you can hear or feel the patient exhale between breaths.
   (c) you can feel the resistance of the chest change as you ventilate the patient.
   (d) you notice the patient's abdomen has become considerably larger.
   (e) the patient's skin color does not improve.

47. All of the following will interfere with your ability to adequately ventilate a patient, except
   (a) removing your mouth from the patient's and releasing closure of the nose between ventilations.
   (b) allowing the nose to remain open while ventilating to allow for passive exhalation.
   (c) keeping the mouth slightly closed to avoid obstruction of the airway.
   (d) maintaining your tight seal over the mouth while taking your next breath in through your nose.
   (e) pushing as hard as you can to acheive a tight seal over the patient's mouth.

48. The rate of mouth-to-mask or mouth-to-mouth artificial respirations for an adult is
   (a) 10 respirations per minute.
   (b) 12 respirations per minute.
   (c) 15 respirations per minute.
   (d) 20 respirations per minute.
   (e) 26 respirations per minute.

49. The rate of mouth-to-mask or mouth-to-mouth artificial respirations for a child is
   (a) 10 respirations per minute.
   (b) 12 respirations per minute.
   (c) 15 respirations per minute.
   (d) 20 respirations per minute.
   (e) 26 respirations per minute.

50. The rate of mouth-to-mask or mouth-to-mouth artificial respirations for an infant is
   (a) 10 respirations per minute.
   (b) 12 respirations per minute.
   (c) 15 respirations per minute.
   (d) 20 respirations per minute.
   (e) 26 respirations per minute.

51. The reasons to use the mouth-to-nose technique of artificial respirations include all of the following, except

    (a) a severe injury in the mouth region.

    (b) a laryngectomy patient.

    (c) when the patient's mouth is larger than the rescuer's mouth.

    (d) when the patient's jaw is wired shut.

    (e) when absent dentures prevent obtaining a tight seal.

52. Which of the following statements regarding mouth-to-nose ventilation is false?

    (a) One hand remains on the patient's forehead at all times.

    (b) The nose is never pinched closed.

    (c) The mouth is never ventilated.

    (d) Your mouth is sealed around the patient's nose only.

    (e) The mouth remains slightly open at all times.

53. Which of the following statements regarding artificial respirations for infants and small children is false?

    (a) An exaggerated head-tilt may obstruct breathing passages.

    (b) Inadequate head-tilt may produce an inadequate airway.

    (c) A seal may be made around both the mouth and nose.

    (d) Use only enough inflation volume to cause the chest to rise.

    (e) Ventilate infants once every 6 seconds.

54. A person who has permanently had all or part of her/his larynx surgically removed is referred to as a _____ patient.

    (a) tracheostomy

    (b) mute

    (c) laryngectomy

    (d) stoma

    (e) cricothyrotomy

55. The _____ is a permanent breathing hole surgically made in a patient's trachea.

    (a) tracheostomy

    (b) mute

    (c) laryngectomy

    (d) stoma

    (e) cricothyrotomy

56. Which of the following statements regarding patients who are "neck breathers" is false?

    (a) If there is no movement of air at the patient's nose and mouth, always check the patient's neck for an opening.

    (b) Those patients whose larynx has been partially removed breathe both through their neck opening, and their nose and mouth.

    (c) Those patients whose complete larynx has been removed breathe only through their neck opening.

    (d) Foreign matter (dried blood, mucous) should be removed from the neck opening with gloved hands and/or suction.

    (e) To perform artificial respiration on a patient with a partially removed larynx, occlude the neck opening with a gloved hand and use mouth-to-mask ventilations.

57. Which of the following statements regarding gastric distention is true?

    (a) Slight distention is common and should be ignored.

    (b) Artificial ventilation rarely causes distention of the abdomen.

    (c) Evacuation of gastric distention with abdominal thrusts is mandatory to allow for adequate ventilation.

    (d) Gastric distention is caused by inadequate volume of ventilations.

    (e) A properly positioned airway will never result in gastric distention.

58. Obstruction of the airway may be caused by all of the following, except

    (a) the epiglottis.

    (b) the patient holding his breath too long and becoming unconscious.

    (c) ingested or inhaled foreign objects.

    (d) damage to the airway from trauma, inhalation of smoke or hot air, or ingested poisons.

    (e) infections, anaphylaxis, allergic reactions, or chronic pulmonary diseases.

59.   You are called to the capital building, where a visiting
Jamaican dignitary is complaining of shortness of breath.
His skin color is much darker than any patient you have
ever seen, but his companions insist that he looks very
pale. You should
  (a) check his nail beds and palms for pallor or cyanosis.
  (b) check the lining of his mouth and eyes for pallor or
        cyanosis.
  (c) document his skin color as being "pale, per report of
        friends."
  (d) Both answers (a) and (b).
  (e) Both answers (a) and (c).

60.   Which of the following statements regarding a partial airway
obstruction is true?
  (a) The patient cannot speak.
  (b) The patient cannot cough.
  (c) Gentle back blows are frequently all that is needed to
        assist the patient.
  (d) All of the above are true.
  (e) None of the above is true.

61.   Which of the following statements regarding a complete
airway obstruction is false?
  (a) The patient cannot speak.
  (b) The patient cannot cough.
  (c) Gentle back blows are frequently all that is needed to
        assist the patient.
  (d) All of the above are false.
  (e) None of the above is false.

62.   Which of the following statements regarding management of
an obstructed airway is true?
  (a) Back blows precede abdominal thrusts on all patients.
  (b) Another name for abdominal thrusts is the "Heinrich
        Maneuver."
  (c) Unless the obstructing object is dislodged with fewer
        thrusts, the EMT should perform 6 to 10 rapid, inward
        and upward abdominal thrusts.
  (d) All of the above are true.
  (e) None of the above is true.

63. Which of the following statements regarding the chest thrust maneuver is true?

    (a) The chest thrust maneuver is used only if abdominal thrusts are ineffective.

    (b) The landmarks for fist placement when one is performing chest thrusts are exactly the same as for performing chest compressions in CPR.

    (c) Unless the obstructing object is dislodged with fewer thrusts, the EMT should perform 6 to 10 rapid, backward chest thrusts.

    (d) All of the above are true.

    (e) None of the above is true.

64. Which of the following statements regarding finger sweeps is false?

    (a) There is little risk of injury when one is performing finger sweeps on an unconscious patient; however, gloves should be worn to prevent contraction of communicable disease.

    (b) Do not perform "blind" finger sweeps on infants or children.

    (c) Turn the patient's head to the side before sweeping (unless spine injury is suspected).

    (d) All of the above are false.

    (e) None of the above is false.

The following four questions concern the same event:

65. You are eating at a restaurant with your family when a nearby commotion catches your attention. You notice a conscious middle-aged man who is sitting in a chair and exhibiting the universal sign of choking. He is cyanotic and quiet with a very distressed expression. You should immediately

    (a) perform 6 to 10 back blows.

    (b) perform 6 to 10 abdominal thrusts.

    (c) ask, "Are you choking? Can you speak? Can you cough?"

    (d) solicit information from bystanders.

    (e) perform finger sweeps and call for help.

66. After the tenth abdominal thrust, the patient's airway status remains unchanged; however, he no longer has his eyes open and does not appear to be making as much effort to breathe as before. You should

(a) perform 6 to 10 back blows.
(b) repeat the 6 to 10 abdominal thrusts.
(c) ask, "Are you choking? Can you speak? Can you cough?"
(d) solicit information from bystanders.
(e) perform finger sweeps and call for help.

67. As you continue with your treatment, the patient becomes unconscious and begins to slide from his chair. You support him to prevent trauma and guide him onto the floor into a supine position. You should immediately

(a) call for help, turn his head to the side, open the airway and perform finger sweeps.
(b) assume the appropriate position and perform 6 to 10 abdominal thrusts, then finger sweeps.
(c) roll him to his side and perform 6 to 10 back blows, then finger sweeps.
(d) call for help, assume the appropriate position, and perform 6 to 10 abdominal thrusts, then finger sweeps.
(e) call for help, roll him to his side, and perform 6 to 10 back blows, then finger sweeps.

68. Your finger sweeps draw some mucous and saliva from the oropharynx, but no large pieces of matter. You should immediately

(a) call for help, turn his head, and repeat the finger sweeps.
(b) call for help, position yourself, and repeat the abdominal thrusts, then the finger sweeps.
(c) call for help, roll the patient to his side, and repeat the back blows, then the finger sweeps.
(d) open the airway and attempt to visualize the matter lodged in the patient's airway.
(e) open the airway and attempt ventilation.

The following three questions concern the same event:

69. A week later, at the same restaurant, you are eating with your family when you hear a commotion coming from the ladies' room. A woman runs out, screaming, "She choked to death! She choked to death!" As you enter the bathroom, you see an obese woman lying on the floor. There is no

apparent trauma, but she is very cyanotic. You should immediately

(a) check for a pulse and call for help.
(b) check for breathing and call for help.
(c) check for level of consciousness and call for help.
(d) perform 6 to 10 chest thrusts and call for help.
(e) perform 6 to 10 back blows and call for help.

70. Your first attempt to ventilate the patient is unsuccessful. You should immediately

(a) perform 6 to 10 chest thrusts, then finger sweeps, and attempt to ventilate again.
(b) perform 6 to 10 abdominal thrusts, then finger sweeps, and attempt to ventilate again.
(c) reposition the airway and attempt to ventilate again.
(d) check for a pulse and attempt to ventilate again.
(e) perform finger sweeps and attempt to ventilate again.

71. Your second attempt to ventilate the patient is also unsuccessful. Using the following, indicate the correct sequence of activities you should perform until ventilation is achieved. (Not all the activities must be used.)

1) Reposition the airway and attempt to ventilate again.
2) Check the patient's pulse.
3) Perform six to ten abdominal thrusts.
4) Perform finger sweeps.
5) Perform six to ten chest thrusts.
6) Perform four slow, firm back blows.
7) Open the airway and attempt to ventilate the patient.
8) Perform four slow, distinct chest thrusts.

(a) 8, 4, 7, 1 and repeat until ventilation is achieved.
(b) 1, 3, 4, 7, 2 and repeat until ventilation is achieved.
(c) 2, 3, 4, 7, 1 and repeat until ventilation is achieved.
(d) 8, 6, 4, 7, 1 and repeat until ventilation is achieved.
(e) 6, 3, 4, 7, 2 and repeat until ventilation is achieved.

72. The heart is a muscular organ approximately the size of

(a) the liver.
(b) a grapefruit.
(c) a man's clenched fist.
(d) a man's open hand.
(e) a tennis ball.

73.   The heart is located in the
   (a) retroperitoneal area of the chest.
   (b) mediastinum, the center of the thoracic cavity.
   (c) retrothoracic area of the chest.
   (d) mediatinum, the sac surrounding the heart.
   (e) the substernal cavity of the chest.

74.   The sac that surrounds the heart is called the
   (a) mediastinum or mediastinal sac.
   (b) cardiac sac.
   (c) pericardium or pericardial sac.
   (d) cardiac membrane.
   (e) cardiac tamponade.

75.   The wall that divides the two upper and two lower chambers
   of the heart is called the
   (a) septum.
   (b) diaphragm.
   (c) cardiac cleavage.
   (d) All of the above.
   (e) None of the above.

76.   A system of _____ keeps the blood moving through the heart
   in the proper direction and prevents backflow.
   (a) two-way valves
   (b) veins and capillaries
   (c) three-way valves
   (d) arteries and capillaries
   (e) one-way valves

77.   The left side of the heart receives _____ and pumps it
   _____.
   (a) blood that has circulated through the body/out to all
        body parts
   (b) blood that has circulated through the body/to the lungs
        to be reoxygenated
   (c) oxygenated blood from the body/to the lungs to be
        exchanged
   (d) oxygenated blood from the lungs/out to all body parts
   (e) deoxygenated blood from the lungs/out to all body parts

78.   The right side of the heart receives _____ and pumps
   it _____.
   (a) blood that has circulated through the body/out to all
        body parts

    (b) blood that has circulated through the body/to the lungs to be reoxygenated

    (c) oxygenated blood from the body/to the lungs to be exchanged

    (d) oxygenated blood from the lungs/out to all body parts

    (e) deoxygenated blood from the lungs/out to all body parts

79. The thick, muscular-walled vessels that carry blood rich in oxygen and other nutrients from the heart to the body cells are called

    (a) veins.

    (b) alveoli.

    (c) arteries.

    (d) lymph glands.

    (e) capillaries.

80. The nonmuscular vessels that carry deoxygenated blood and waste products from the body cells to the heart are called

    (a) veins.

    (b) alveoli.

    (c) arteries.

    (d) lymph glands.

    (e) capillaries.

81. The very, very thin-walled vessels through which oxygen and carbon dioxide, nutrients, and waste materials are exchanged within the body cells or lungs are called

    (a) veins.

    (b) alveoli.

    (c) arteries.

    (d) lymph glands.

    (e) capillaries.

82. Artificial circulation is accomplished by compression of the sternum, which

    (a) compresses the heart to pump the blood through the body.

    (b) causes pressure changes in the thoracic cavity to circulate the blood to the body.

    (c) causes pressure changes in the thoracic cavity to circulate the blood to the lungs.

    (d) All of the above.

    (e) None of the above.

83. When performed correctly, with 90 to 100 percent oxygen supplementation, CPR is _____ as effective as the action of the normal, healthy heart.

 (a) 63 to 75 percent
 (b) 45 to 53 percent
 (c) 25 to 33 percent
 (d) 10 to 20 percent
 (e) 90 to 100 percent

84. After effectively ventilating an obese patient who was not breathing, you should immediately

 (a) perform 6 to 10 abdominal thrusts.
 (b) perform 4 slow chest thrusts.
 (c) check for a radial pulse.
 (d) perform finger sweeps.
 (e) check for a carotid pulse.

85. The amount of time required to determine pulselessness is

 (a) the time it takes to say "capillary refill."
 (b) 1 to 3 seconds.
 (c) 3 to 5 seconds.
 (d) the amount of time you can comfortably hold your own breath.
 (e) 5 to 10 seconds.

86. If no pulse is present, you should immediately

 (a) begin chest compressions and perform ACLS.
 (b) activate the EMS system (requesting ACLS) and begin chest compressions.
 (c) reposition the airway and repeat ventilations.
 (d) perform CPR for one minute and then activate the EMS system, requesting ACLS.
 (e) activate the EMS system (requesting ACLS), repeat ventilations, and begin chest compressions.

87. If the patient in cardiopulmonary arrest is found in a chair,

 (a) do not delay performance of CPR. Perform CPR for one minute and then move the patient to a firm surface.
 (b) delay CPR until the patient is in the ambulance.

    (c) call the medical examiner.

    (d) delay CPR until the patient is on a firm surface, such as the ground or a spine board.

    (e) delay CPR, remove all of the patient's clothing, move the patient to a firm surface, then start CPR.

88.   If the patient in cardiopulmonary arrest is found in a bed,

    (a) do not delay performance of CPR. Perform CPR for one minute and then move the patient to a firm surface.

    (b) delay CPR until the patient is in the ambulance.

    (c) call the medical examiner.

    (d) delay CPR until the patient is on a firm surface, such as the ground or a spine board.

    (e) delay CPR, remove all of the patient's clothing, move the patient to a firm surface, then start CPR.

89.   If the patient in cardiopulmonary arrest is found on a flight of stairs,

    (a) do not delay performance of CPR. Perform CPR for one minute and then move the patient to a firm surface.

    (b) delay CPR until the patient is in the ambulance.

    (c) call the medical examiner.

    (d) delay CPR until the patient is on a firm surface, such as the ground or a spine board.

    (e) delay CPR, remove all of the patient's clothing, move the patient to a firm surface, then start CPR.

90.   Which of the following statements regarding performance of CPR is false?

    (a) If the mechanism of injury suggests spine injury, chest compressions must be delayed until the patient is secured to a backboard. However, ventilations may be started, using the modified jaw-thrust maneuver, and continued until spinal immobilization allows for initiation of chest compressions.

    (b) Elevation of the lower extremities, while keeping the rest of the body horizontal, may promote venous return and aid circulation of blood during CPR.

    (c) Pneumatic counter-pressure device trousers (PASG or MAST) may assist in venous return and aid circulation of blood during CPR.

    (d) All of the above are false.

    (e) None of the above is false.

91. The location of hand placement for chest compressions on an adult is

(a) the upper third of the sternum, just below the suprasternal notch.
(b) the lower half of the sternum, just above the substernal notch.
(c) immediately on top of the substernal notch.
(d) immediately below the substernal notch.
(e) the middle of the sternum, on the intermammary (nipple) line.

92. For single-rescuer CPR on an adult, compress the sternum approximately

(a) 0 to ½ inch.
(b) ½ to 1 inch.
(c) 1 to 1½ inches.
(d) 1½ to 2 inches.
(e) 2 to 2½ inches.

93. For one- or two-rescuer CPR on a child, compress the sternum approximately

(a) 0 to ½ inch.
(b) ½ to 1 inch.
(c) 1 to 1½ inches.
(d) 1½ to 2 inches.
(e) 2 to 2½ inches.

94. For one- or two-rescuer CPR on an infant, compress the sternum approximately

(a) 0 to ½ inch.
(b) ½ to 1 inch.
(c) 1 to 1½ inches.
(d) 1½ to 2 inches.
(e) 2 to 2½ inches.

95. The standard age-range definition of "a child" is

(a) 6 months to 18 years old.
(b) 1 year to 18 years old.
(c) birth to 1 year old.
(d) birth to 2 years old.
(e) birth to 6 months old.

96. The standard age-range definition of "an infant" is

(a) 6 months to 18 years old.

(b) 1 year to 18 years old.

(c) birth to 1 year old.

(d) birth to 2 years old.

(e) birth to 6 months old.

97. For two-rescuer CPR on an adult, compress the sternum approximately

(a) 0 to ½ inch.

(b) ½ to 1 inch.

(c) 1 to 1½ inches.

(d) 1½ to 2 inches.

(e) 2 to 2½ inches.

98. For single-rescuer CPR on an adult, compress the sternum at a rate of approximately

(a) 100 to 120 times per minute.

(b) 80 to 100 times per minute.

(c) at least 100 times per minute.

(d) 60 to 80 times per minute.

(e) 40 to 60 times per minute.

99. For one- or two-rescuer CPR on a child, compress the sternum at a rate of approximately

(a) 100 to 120 times per minute.

(b) 80 to 100 times per minute.

(c) at least 100 times per minute.

(d) 60 to 80 times per minute.

(e) 40 to 60 times per minute.

100. For one- or two-rescuer CPR on an infant, compress the sternum at a rate of approximately

(a) 100 to 120 times per minute.

(b) 80 to 100 times per minute.

(c) at least 100 times per minute.

(d) 60 to 80 times per minute.

(e) 40 to 60 times per minute.

101. For two-rescuer CPR on an adult, compress the sternum at a rate of approximately

(a) 100 to 120 times per minute.

(b) 80 to 100 times per minute.

(c) at least 100 times per minute.

(d) 60 to 80 times per minute.

(e) 40 to 60 times per minute.

102. The positioning of the hands for chest compression of an adult is

    (a) the heel of each hand, side by side, on the sternum.

    (b) the heel of one hand in the middle of the sternum.

    (c) the tips of the index and middle fingers in the middle of the sternum.

    (d) Any of the above.

    (e) None of the above.

103. After beginning CPR, the EMT should recheck for return of the patient's pulse

    (a) after one minute, then every few minutes.

    (b) after each cycle of compressions/ventilation, before beginning the next cycle.

    (c) after the first 5 cycles of compressions/ventilation, then every 10 cycles.

    (d) after each minute of compressions/ventilations, until the return of pulse or respirations.

    (e) after each 5-minute period of compressions/ventilations.

104. The most reliable sign of effective performance of CPR is

    (a) improvement of skin color.

    (b) constriction of pupils to light.

    (c) observation of chest rise with ventilation and the presence of a carotid pulse during compressions.

    (d) strict adherence to the appropriate measurement of chest compressions and the appropriate number of ventilations.

    (e) using the appropriate counting method for compression and ventilation timing.

105. The xyphoid process is located

    (a) at the distal end of the sternum.

    (b) immediately above a portion of the liver.

    (c) at the meeting of the right and left costal margins.

    (d) All of the above.

    (e) None of the above.

106. Which of the following is a possible complication of correctly performed chest compression?

    (a) Fractured ribs.

    (b) Fractured or flailed sternum.

    (c) Lacerations of the liver, spleen, lungs, or heart.

(d) All of the above.

(e) None of the above.

107. Which of the following is a possible complication of incorrectly performed chest compression?

    (a) Fractured ribs.

    (b) Fractured or flailed sternum.

    (c) Lacerations of the liver, spleen, lungs, or heart.

    (d) All of the above.

    (e) None of the above.

108. Which of the following frequently occurs when chest compression is performed correctly?

    (a) Fractured ribs.

    (b) Fractured or flailed sternum.

    (c) Lacerations of the liver, spleen, lungs, or heart.

    (d) All of the above.

    (e) None of the above.

109. While performing chest compressions, if you hear or feel a "cracking" or "crunching" sensation, you should

    (a) disregard the sensation and continue CPR (it is not unusual to separate cartilage when compressing the chest).

    (b) stop CPR (fractured ribs may produce a pneumothorax if CPR is continued).

    (c) reassess your location of hand placement and consider adjusting the depth of your compressions, but continue CPR.

    (d) move to a different (unfractured) portion of the sternum and continue CPR.

    (e) continue compressions in the same location but at half the previous depth.

110. Your patient is emaciated, has labored respirations, and a very weak carotid pulse. He is in the terminal stages of an incurable condition. The family members indicate that they do not want any CPR done should he suffer a cardiopulmonary arrest while in your care. Just as they say this, the patient arrests. You should

(a) honor the family's wishes and allow the patient to expire with dignity.

(b) assume that the patient would want CPR and perform it.

(c) delay CPR for no longer than 10 minutes to allow the family time to locate written/signed "Do Not Resuscitate" orders (or to contact the patient's physician by phone for verbal orders).

(d) not delay CPR unless a clearly documented and notarized "Living Will" or physician's signed orders are present.

(e) begin CPR. When sufficient help arrives, have CPR continued while you contact your physician advisor by phone to request "Do Not Resucitate" orders on behalf of the family's wishes.

111. Which of the following statements is not an acceptable reason for terminating CPR?

(a) Terminate CPR when the patient's husband states that he wants no more damage done to his wife's body.

(b) Terminate CPR when you are too exhausted to continue.

(c) Terminate CPR when another team of EMTs assumes care of the patient.

(d) Terminate chest compressions when the patient has the return of his own pulse, but continue rescue breathing or ventilations as needed.

(e) Terminate CPR when the coroner pronounces the patient dead.

112. The ratio of chest compressions to ventilations for one-rescuer CPR on an adult is

(a) 15 compressions alternated with 2 ventilations.

(b) 10 compressions alternated with 2 ventilations.

(c) 15 compressions alternated with 1 ventilation.

(d) 7 compressions alternated with 1 ventilation.

(e) 5 compressions alternated with 1 ventilation.

113. The ratio of chest compressions to ventilations for two-rescuer CPR on an adult is

(a) 15 compressions alternated with 2 ventilations.
(b) 10 compressions alternated with 2 ventilations.
(c) 15 compressions alternated with 1 ventilation.
(d) 7 compressions alternated with 1 ventilation.
(e) 5 compressions alternated with 1 ventilation.

114. The ratio of chest compressions to ventilations for one-rescuer CPR on a child is

(a) 15 compressions alternated with 2 ventilations.
(b) 10 compressions alternated with 2 ventilations.
(c) 15 compressions alternated with 1 ventilation.
(d) 7 compressions alternated with 1 ventilation.
(e) 5 compressions alternated with 1 ventilation.

115. The ratio of chest compressions to ventilations for two-rescuer CPR on a child is

(a) 15 compressions alternated with 2 ventilations.
(b) 10 compressions alternated with 2 ventilations.
(c) 15 compressions alternated with 1 ventilation.
(d) 7 compressions alternated with 1 ventilation.
(e) 5 compressions alternated with 1 ventilation.

116. The ratio of chest compressions to ventilations for one-rescuer CPR on an infant is

(a) 15 compressions alternated with 2 ventilations.
(b) 10 compressions alternated with 2 ventilations.
(c) 15 compressions alternated with 1 ventilation.
(d) 7 compressions alternated with 1 ventilation.
(e) 5 compressions alternated with 1 ventilation.

117. The ratio of chest compressions to ventilations for two-rescuer CPR on an infant is

(a) 15 compressions alternated with 2 ventilations.
(b) 10 compressions alternated with 2 ventilations.
(c) 15 compressions alternated with 1 ventilation.
(d) 7 compressions alternated with 1 ventilation.
(e) 5 compressions alternated with 1 ventilation.

118. Which of the following statements regarding interruption of CPR is true?

    (a) CPR should never be interrupted for more than 5 seconds.

    (b) CPR may be interrupted for 15 to 30 seconds in cases of emergency moves or other special circumstances.

    (c) CPR should never be interrupted for more than 7 seconds.

    (d) CPR should never be interrupted for more than 15 to 30 seconds.

    (e) CPR may be interrupted only for the lone rescuer in a secluded location to go for help (and only after having performed CPR for at least one minute).

119. When making the transition between one-rescuer and two-rescuer CPR, a pulse check is made

    (a) by the first rescuer, while the second rescuer locates the correct chest compression site.

    (b) by the second rescuer, as the first continues chest compressions until she/he is told to stop.

    (c) by the second rescuer, while the first rescuer performs rescue breathing only.

    (d) only after the first full minute of two-person CPR.

    (e) only after the first two-person compression/ventilation cycle is completed.

120. The amount of time allowed for periodic checks to determine if the patient's pulse has returned is

    (a) the time it takes to say, "capillary refill."

    (b) 1 to 3 seconds.

    (c) 5 seconds.

    (d) the amount of time you can comfortably hold your own breath.

    (e) 5 to 10 seconds.

121. Which of the following statements regarding two-rescuer CPR is true?

    (a) Deliver one compression per second.

    (b) Do not disrupt the compressor's count. If the ventilator misses a ventilation, she/he should wait for the next cycle before ventilating.

    (c) The compressor should pause 1 to 1½ seconds to allow for the ventilation.

(d) The ventilator should deliver the ventilations on the downstroke of every tenth compression.

(e) The ventilator should deliver the ventilations on the upstroke of every tenth compression.

122. To determine pulselessness when the patient is an infant, the EMT should feel for the

    (a) brachial pulse.

    (b) radial pulse.

    (c) carotid pulse.

    (d) femoral pulse.

    (e) pediatric pulse.

123. To determine pulselessness when the patient is a child, the EMT should feel for the

    (a) brachial pulse.

    (b) radial pulse.

    (c) carotid pulse.

    (d) femoral pulse.

    (e) pediatric pulse.

124. The location of the chest compression site on an infant is

    (a) the same as that of an adult.

    (b) immediately on and one finger width below the intermammary (nipple) line.

    (c) two finger widths below the left nipple.

    (d) two finger widths below the intermammary (nipple) line.

    (e) the same as that of a child.

125. The location of the chest compression site on a child is

    (a) the same as that of an adult.

    (b) immediately on and one finger width below the intermammary (nipple) line.

    (c) two finger widths below the left nipple.

    (d) two finger widths below the intermammary (nipple) line.

    (e) the same as that of an infant.

126. The _____ can be used to maintain an open airway on deeply unresponsive patients.

    (a) oropharyngeal airway

    (b) nasopharyngeal airway

    (c) laryngeal airway

    (d) Both answers (a) and (b).

    (e) Both answers (b) and (c).

127. The _____ may be used on a conscious patient who cannot maintain an open airway.

    (a) oropharyngeal airway

    (b) nasopharyngeal airway

    (c) laryngeal airway

    (d) Both answers (a) and (b).

    (e) Both answers (b) and (c).

128. The _____ may be used on an unconscious patient who continues to have a gag reflex.

    (a) oropharyngeal airway

    (b) nasopharyngeal airway

    (c) laryngeal airway

    (d) Both answers (a) and (b).

    (e) Both answers (b) and (c).

129. The _____ can force the tongue back into the pharynx and cause an obstruction.

    (a) oropharyngeal airway

    (b) nasopharyngeal airway

    (c) laryngeal airway

    (d) Both answers (a) and (b).

    (e) Both answers (b) and (c).

130. Insertion of the _____ may cause vomiting or spasm of the vocal cords.

    (a) oropharyngeal airway

    (b) nasopharyngeal airway

    (c) laryngeal airway

    (d) Both answers (a) and (b).

    (e) Both answers (b) and (c).

131. Lubrication is required to insert the _____.

    (a) oropharyngeal airway

    (b) nasopharyngeal airway

    (c) laryngeal airway

    (d) Both answers (a) and (b).

    (e) Both answers (b) and (c).

132. The _____ is made of hard, inflexible plastic.

    (a) oropharyngeal airway

    (b) nasopharyngeal airway

(c) laryngeal airway
(d) Both answers (a) and (b).
(e) Both answers (b) and (c).

133. The _____ is made of soft, flexible plastic or rubber.
(a) oropharyngeal airway
(b) nasopharyngeal airway
(c) laryngeal airway
(d) Both answers (a) and (b).
(e) Both answers (b) and (c).

134. The _____ may cause hemorrhage even when properly sized and inserted.
(a) oropharyngeal airway
(b) nasopharyngeal airway
(c) laryngeal airway
(d) Both answers (a) and (b).
(e) Both answers (b) and (c).

135. The _____ will not perform effectively if an inappropriate size has been selected.
(a) oropharyngeal airway
(b) nasopharyngeal airway
(c) laryngeal airway
(d) Both answers (a) and (b).
(e) Both answers (b) and (c).

136. Size selection of the oropharyngeal airway is accomplished by externally comparing it to the patient's body and selecting an airway that measures from
(a) the front of the nose to the tip of the earlobe.
(b) the corner of the mouth to the tip of the earlobe.
(c) the center of the mouth to the angle of the jaw.
(d) Either answers (a) or (b).
(e) Either answers (b) or (c).

137. Size selection of the nasopharyngeal airway is accomplished by externally comparing it to the patient's body and selecting an airway that measures from
(a) the front of the nose to the tip of the earlobe.
(b) the corner of the mouth to the tip of the earlobe.
(c) the center of the mouth to the angle of the jaw.
(d) Either answers (a) or (b).
(e) Either answers (b) or (c).

138. The diameter of the nasopharyngeal airway should be
  - (a) the same size as the patient's nostril.
  - (b) the same size as the diameter of the patient's little finger.
  - (c) slightly smaller than the patient's nostril.
  - (d) Both answers (a) and (b).
  - (e) Both answers (b) and (c).

139. Which of the following statements regarding airway adjunct lubrication is true?
  - (a) Water-based lubricants are preferred; however, mineral oil is acceptable.
  - (b) Either petroleum jelly or vaseline is the preferred lubricant because of their viscosity.
  - (c) Only water-based lubricants may be used as airway lubricants.
  - (d) Either mineral oil or sterile water can be used as an airway lubricant.
  - (e) Either Normal Saline or sterile water may be used as an airway lubricant.

140. Which of the following statements regarding insertion of an oropharyngeal airway is true?
  - (a) Insert the airway with the tip facing downward and gently slide it over and behind the tongue.
  - (b) The use of a tongue blade will aid in insertion of the airway.
  - (c) Lubricate the airway well, so that it will slide gently behind the tongue with a minimum of trauma.
  - (d) Hyperflexion of the neck is required for proper insertion of the airway.
  - (e) Hyperextension of the neck is required for proper insertion of the airway.

141. Rigid pharyngeal suction tips
  - (a) are better than flexible suction devices when one is suctioning the pharynx or large pieces of vomitus.
  - (b) may induce vomiting if used on a conscious patient.
  - (c) may induce vomiting if used on an unconscious patient who still has a gag reflex.
  - (d) All of the above.
  - (e) None of the above.

142. Suction is employed to remove fluids and/or obstructive materials from the
   (a) mouth and pharynx.
   (b) nose and mouth.
   (c) nose, mouth, and stoma.
   (d) nose, pharynx, and stoma.
   (e) mouth, pharynx and stoma.

143. Never suction a breathing patient
   (a) longer than 15 seconds.
   (b) longer than you can comfortably hold your own breath.
   (c) longer than 5 seconds.
   (d) Both answers (a) and (b).
   (e) Both answers (b) and (c).

144. Never suction a nonbreathing patient
   (a) longer than 15 seconds.
   (b) longer than you can comfortably hold your own breath.
   (c) longer than 5 seconds.
   (d) Both answers (a) and (b).
   (e) Both answers (b) and (c).

145. Suction is applied
   (a) only while withdrawing the catheter.
   (b) only while inserting the catheter.
   (c) only while the catheter is stationary.
   (d) only after the patient has been ventilated for at least 10 minutes.
   (e) only with an oropharyngeal or nasopharyngeal airway in place.

146. The maximum depth of suction catheter insertion is
   (a) the distance between the tip of the catheter and the hole in the catheter's side.
   (b) equal to the distance from the corner of the patient's mouth to the lobe of the patient's ear.
   (c) equal to the distance from the center of the patient's mouth to the angle of the patient's jaw.
   (d) Both answers (a) and (b).
   (e) Both answers (b) and (c)

147. A pocket-mask with an oxygen inlet and a one-way valve, used with oxygen run at 10 LPM, will provide the nonbreathing patient with approximately _____ during mouth-to-mask resuscitation.

    (a) 10 percent oxygen
    (b) 50 percent oxygen
    (c) 15 percent oxygen
    (d) 80 percent oxygen
    (e) 90 percent oxygen

148. A pocket-mask with an oxygen inlet and a one-way valve, used with oxygen run at 15 LPM, will provide the nonbreathing patient with approximately _____ during mouth-to-mask resuscitation.

    (a) 10 percent oxygen
    (b) 50 percent oxygen
    (c) 15 percent oxygen
    (d) 80 percent oxygen
    (e) 90 percent oxygen

149. Which of the following statements is false?

    (a) Some adult pocket-masks may be inverted for use on small children and infants.
    (b) When using either the pocket-mask or the bag-valve-mask, an oropharyngeal or nasopharyngeal airway should be in place.
    (c) Better ventilation volumes are delivered by direct mouth-to-mask resuscitation than by the bag-valve-mask device.
    (d) All of the above are false.
    (e) None of the above is false.

150. With proper operation and a 15 LPM oxygen flow rate, the bag-valve-mask device will deliver a concentration of

    (a) 35 to 40 percent oxygen.
    (b) 50 percent oxygen.
    (c) 60 to 70 percent oxygen.
    (d) more than 90 percent oxygen.
    (e) 100 percent oxygen.

151. With proper operation, a 15 LPM oxygen flow rate, and an oxygen reservoir, the bag-valve-mask device will deliver a concentration of

    (a) 35 to 40 percent oxygen.
    (b) 50 percent oxygen.

    (c)   60 to 70 percent oxygen.

    (d)   more than 90 percent oxygen.

    (e)   100 percent oxygen.

152. Which of the following statements regarding oxygen administration is false?

    (a)   If you are unsure whether or not the patient requires supplemental oxygen, do not administer it.

    (b)   All patients requiring pulmonary or cardiopulmonary resuscitation should receive oxygen as soon as it is available.

    (c)   Do not delay resuscitation to obtain oxygen for the patient.

    (d)   All of the above are false.

    (e)   None of the above is false.

153. Patients who have a decreased level of oxygen in their body tissues are said to be

    (a)   anoxic.

    (b)   hypoxia.

    (c)   hypoxic.

    (d)   hypoxemic.

    (e)   apnic.

154. The finding of insufficient oxygen levels within the patient's blood is called

    (a)   anoxia.

    (b)   hypoxia.

    (c)   hypoxic.

    (d)   hypoxemia.

    (e)   apnea.

155. The finding of insufficient oxygen levels within the patient's body tissues is called

    (a)   anoxia.

    (b)   hypoxia.

    (c)   hypoxic.

    (d)   hypoxemia.

    (e)   apnea.

156. The absence of oxygen within the body tissues is called

    (a) anoxia.

    (b) hypoxia.

    (c) hypoxic.

    (d) hypoxemia.

    (e) apnea.

157. Which of the following statements regarding oxygen is false?

    (a) Oxygen supports combustion and contributes to fire hazard.

    (b) Oxygen is a drug.

    (c) The combination of petroleum products with oxygen will cause an explosion.

    (d) Oxygen is usually supplied as a compressed gas.

    (e) EMS oxygen cylinders are specially equipped with O-rings that prevent them from becoming missiles if they are dropped or punctured.

158. Excessively prolonged administration of high concentrations of oxygen may cause all of the following, except

    (a) lung tissue destruction.

    (b) atelectasis.

    (c) retrolental fibroplasia in infants.

    (d) hypoxic drive.

    (e) respiratory depression.

159. The _____ is portable and contains approximately 350 liters of oxygen.

    (a) D cylinder

    (b) E cylinder

    (c) G cylinder

    (d) H cylinder

    (e) M cylinder

160. The _____ is portable and contains approximately 625 liters of oxygen.

    (a) D cylinder

    (b) E cylinder

    (c) G cylinder

    (d) H cylinder

    (e) M cylinder

161. The _____ is portable and contains approximately 3000 liters of oxygen.
 (a) D cylinder
 (b) E cylinder
 (c) G cylinder
 (d) H cylinder
 (e) M cylinder

162. The _____ is a nonportable cylinder, and contains approximately 5300 liters of oxygen.
 (a) D cylinder
 (b) E cylinder
 (c) G cylinder
 (d) H cylinder
 (e) M cylinder

163. The _____ is a nonportable cylinder, and contains approximately 6900 liters of oxygen.
 (a) D cylinder
 (b) E cylinder
 (c) G cylinder
 (d) H cylinder
 (e) M cylinder

164. The guidelines for oxygen flow when a nasal cannula is used are
 (a) a minimum of 8 LPM to a maximum of 15 LPM.
 (b) a minimum of 1 LPM to a maximum of 6 LPM.
 (c) a minimum of 6 LPM to a maximum of 10 LPM.
 (d) a minimum of 10 LPM to a maximum of 15 LPM.
 (e) a minimum of 4 LPM to a maximum of 8 LPM.

165. The guidelines for oxygen flow when a simple face mask is used are
 (a) a minimum of 8 LPM to a maximum of 15 LPM.
 (b) a minimum of 1 LPM to a maximum of 6 LPM.
 (c) a minimum of 6 LPM to a maximum of 10 LPM.
 (d) a minimum of 10 LPM to a maximum of 15 LPM.
 (e) a minimum of 4 LPM to a maximum of 8 LPM.

166. The guidelines for oxygen flow when a partial rebreather mask is used are

    (a) a minimum of 8 LPM to a maximum of 15 LPM.
    (b) a minimum of 1 LPM to a maximum of 6 LPM.
    (c) a minimum of 6 LPM to a maximum of 10 LPM.
    (d) a minimum of 10 LPM to a maximum of 15 LPM.
    (e) a minimum of 4 LPM to a maximum of 8 LPM.

167. The guidelines for oxygen flow when a nonrebreather mask is used are

    (a) a minimum of 8 LPM to a maximum of 15 LPM.
    (b) a minimum of 1 LPM to a maximum of 6 LPM.
    (c) a minimum of 6 LPM to a maximum of 10 LPM.
    (d) a minimum of 10 LPM to a maximum of 15 LPM.
    (e) a minimum of 4 LPM to a maximum of 8 LPM.

168. The guidelines for oxygen flow when a venturi mask is used are

    (a) a minimum of 8 LPM to a maximum of 15 LPM.
    (b) a minimum of 1 LPM to a maximum of 6 LPM.
    (c) a minimum of 6 LPM to a maximum of 10 LPM.
    (d) a minimum of 10 LPM to a maximum of 15 LPM.
    (e) a minimum of 4 LPM to a maximum of 8 LPM.

169. With an appropriate liter flow of oxygen, the nasal cannula will deliver

    (a) 24 to 44 percent oxygen.
    (b) in excess of 60 percent oxygen.
    (c) 10, 20, 30, or 40 percent oxygen.
    (d) 35 to 60 percent oxygen.
    (e) 24, 28, 35, or 40 percent oxygen.

170. With an appropriate liter flow of oxygen, the simple face mask will deliver

    (a) 24 to 44 percent oxygen.
    (b) in excess of 60 percent oxygen.
    (c) 10, 20, 30, or 40 percent oxygen.
    (d) 35 to 60 percent oxygen.
    (e) 24, 28, 35, or 40 percent oxygen.

171. With an appropriate liter flow of oxygen, the partial rebreather mask will deliver

    (a) 24 to 44 percent oxygen.
    (b) in excess of 60 percent oxygen.

    (c) 10, 20, 30, or 40 percent oxygen.
    (d) 35 to 60 percent oxygen.
    (e) 24, 28, 35, or 40 percent oxygen.

172. With an appropriate liter flow of oxygen, the non-rebreather mask will deliver
    (a) 24 to 44 percent oxygen.
    (b) in excess of 60 percent oxygen.
    (c) 10, 20, 30, or 40 percent oxygen.
    (d) 35 to 60 percent oxygen.
    (e) 24, 28, 35, or 40 percent oxygen.

173. With an appropriate liter flow of oxygen, the venturi mask will deliver
    (a) 24 to 44 percent oxygen.
    (b) in excess of 60 percent oxygen.
    (c) 10, 20, 30, or 40 percent oxygen.
    (d) 35 to 60 percent oxygen.
    (e) 24, 28, 35, or 40 percent oxygen.

174. Which of the following statements regarding oxygen administration is false?
    (a) For all oxygen masks equipped with bags, the oxygen liter flow must be set at least high enough to prevent complete collapse of the bag.
    (b) If a venturi mask is set at too high a liter flow of oxygen, the patient will receive too high a concentration.
    (c) A pediatric- or infant-size mask should be used for a stoma.
    (d) Simple face masks and partial rebreather masks allow the patient to breathe some room air no matter how tightly they are applied.
    (e) A nonrebreather mask will not deliver 100 percent oxygen even when set at 15 LPM.

175. Which of the following statements is true?

  (a) A demand valve resuscitator will deliver 100 percent oxygen despite a poorly sealed mask.
  (b) Both the bag-valve-mask device and the demand valve resuscitator can be used to assist a breathing patient's respirations.
  (c) The demand valve resuscitator will deliver a ventilation only when manually triggered by the EMT.
  (d) Both the bag-valve-mask device and the demand valve resuscitator have child- and pediatric-sized masks for use on a variety of patients.
  (e) The oxygen source for the demand valve resuscitator should be run at 15 LPM at all times.

176. A structural defect or functional abnormality that a patient is born with is called a

  (a) natant abnormality.
  (b) congenerous abnormality.
  (c) congenital anomaly.
  (d) congestive anomaly.
  (e) latent anomaly.

177. A problem that occurs suddenly or develops rapidly is called

  (a) episodic.
  (b) clonic.
  (c) chronic.
  (d) tonic.
  (e) acute.

178. A problem that persists over a prolonged period of time is called

  (a) episodic.
  (b) clonic.
  (c) chronic.
  (d) tonic.
  (e) acute.

179. A problem that fluctuates, occurring or causing difficulty only at certain times, is called

  (a) episodic.
  (b) clonic.
  (c) chronic.

(d) tonic.

(e) acute.

180. An old complaint that suddenly becomes more severe than before can be said to be

(a) episodic.

(b) clonic.

(c) chronic.

(d) tonic.

(e) acute.

181. Any substance that interferes with normal physiologic functions is a

(a) toxin.

(b) poison.

(c) bacteria.

(d) venom.

(e) virus.

182. A poisonous substance that is excreted by some animals and insects and is transmitted by bites or stings is a

(a) toxin.

(b) poison.

(c) bacteria.

(d) venom.

(e) virus.

183. A poisonous substance of plant or animal origin is a

(a) toxin.

(b) poison.

(c) bacteria.

(d) venom.

(e) virus.

184. When an entire body system reacts adversely to a poison, it is called

(a) an inhaled reaction.

(b) a systemic reaction.

(c) a localized reaction.

(d) a medium reaction.

(e) a small reaction.

185. When only a small portion of the body reacts adversely to a poison, it is called

    (a) an inhaled reaction.
    (b) a systemic reaction.
    (c) a localized reaction.
    (d) a medium reaction.
    (e) a small reaction.

186. Poisons that cause harm to the entire body are

    (a) inhaled poisons.
    (b) systemic poisons.
    (c) ingested poisons.
    (d) injected poisons.
    (e) absorbed poisons.

187. Poisons that harm the patient by being swallowed are

    (a) inhaled poisons.
    (b) systemic poisons.
    (c) ingested poisons.
    (d) injected poisons.
    (e) absorbed poisons.

188. Poisons that harm the patient by being breathed into the lungs are

    (a) inhaled poisons.
    (b) systemic poisons.
    (c) ingested poisons.
    (d) injected poisons.
    (e) absorbed poisons.

189. Poisons that harm the patient by entering the body through the skin, skin openings, or mucous membranes are

    (a) inhaled poisons.
    (b) systemic poisons.
    (c) ingested poisons.
    (d) injected poisons.
    (e) absorbed poisons.

190. Poisons that harm the patient when he has been bitten, stung, or stuck with an object are

    (a) inhaled poisons.
    (b) systemic poisons.

(c) ingested poisons.

(d) injected poisons.

(e) absorbed poisons.

191. Which of the following statements regarding ingested poisoning is false?

    (a) Signs and symptoms are variable, depending on the substance ingested.

    (b) The best treatment in most cases is to dilute the substance and induce vomiting.

    (c) Dilution is best accomplished with soda water or juices, as you can rarely get a patient to drink activated charcoal.

    (d) Vomiting is typically induced with syrup of ipecac.

    (e) Ipecac will not work if given at the same time as activated charcoal.

192. Signs or symptoms of systemic poisoning include

    (a) nausea, vomiting, diarrhea, and/or abdominal pain.

    (b) dilation or constriction of pupils, abnormal respirations, seizures, and/or unconsciousness.

    (c) excessive salivation, runny nose, teary eyes, and/or diaphoresis.

    (d) All of the above.

    (e) None of the above.

193. Vomiting should be induced only if

    (a) the conscious patient does not have a gag reflex.

    (b) a petroleum product was ingested.

    (c) an acid or alkali was ingested.

    (d) all of the above have occurred.

    (e) none of the above has occurred.

194. Vomiting should be induced when

    (a) the patient is pregnant, to avoid poisoning of the fetus.

    (b) the patient has a history of heart disease, to avoid cardiac toxicity.

    (c) the patient has ingested a corrosive chemical, to avoid internal bleeding and shock.

    (d) All of the above.

    (e) None of the above.

195. Drugs that prevent vomiting are called
  (a) antiepileptics.
  (b) antibiotics.
  (c) antiemetics.
  (d) antianemics.
  (e) antidiuretics.

196. Which of the following statements regarding ingestion of poisonous plants is false?
  (a) Immediate transport to the emergency room is critical, so that an antidote to the plant poison can be administered without delay.
  (b) A lethal ingestion of poisonous plants can occur in children even if only small pieces were ingested.
  (c) Ingestion of poisonous plants can cause gastro-intestinal disorders.
  (d) Ingestion of poisonous plants can cause nervous system disorders.
  (e) Ingestion of poisonous plants can cause circulatory collapse.

197. The primary concern when one is presented with a victim of an inhaled poison is
  (a) rapid oxygenation of the patient.
  (b) protection from aspiration of vomitus.
  (c) contacting the Poison Control Center for instructions.
  (d) immediately determining the substance inhaled.
  (e) removal of the patient from the source of inhalation, only after ensuring rescuer safety.

198. Which of the following statements regarding absorbed poisons is false?
  (a) Self-protection from contamination takes precedence over patient care.
  (b) Removing the patient from the source and decontamination of the patient must occur before wound treatment can be accomplished.
  (c) Absorbed poisons cannot cause anaphylactic shock unless ingestion or inhalation has occurred.
  (d) All of the above are false.
  (e) None of the above is false.

199. Identification of a black widow spider can be made from the patient's description of observing
- (a) a "fiddle" shape on the top of the spider, behind its eyes.
- (b) black and red bands at the junction of the legs and body parts.
- (c) a yellowish-orange hourglass shape, underneath its largest body segment.
- (d) All of the above.
- (e) Nonc of the above.

200. Identification of a brown recluse spider can be made from the patient's description of observing
- (a) a "fiddle" shape on the top of the spider, behind its eyes.
- (b) black and red bands at the junction of the legs and body parts.
- (c) a yellowish-orange hourglass shape, underneath its largest body segment.
- (d) All of the above.
- (e) None of the above.

201. Which of the following statements regarding spider bites is true?
- (a) Spider bites frequently lead to death.
- (b) Application of ice to the site is mandatory to prevent systemic envenomation.
- (c) Antivenoms are available for black widow spiders only.
- (d) Identification of the specific spider is not important.
- (e) Be very careful during your attempts to capture the insect sample; collect it in a glass jar, pierce holes in the lid, and transport it to the emergency room with the patient.

202. Which of the following statements regarding treatment of bee, wasp, and ant stings is false?
- (a) Use a credit card (or similar object) to carefully scrape away the stinger and venom sac.
- (b) If a credit card is not available, with gloved hands, gently squeeze the stinger and/or venom sac from the site and wipe it away with a clean cloth or sterile 4 X 4.
- (c) Before removal of stinger and venom sac, place a constricting band above the injury, only if it is on an extremity.
- (d) Be alert for signs and symptoms of anaphylaxis.
- (e) You may assist the patient to use her/his bee sting injection kit.

203. Venomous snake species commonly found in the United States include the

    (a) rattlesnake, coral snake, and boa constrictor.

    (b) rattlesnake, cottonmouth, copperhead, and coral snake.

    (c) asp, pit viper, rattlesnake, and water moccasin.

    (d) All of the above.

    (e) None of the above.

204. The two types of poisonous snakes are

    (a) pit vipers and neurotoxic snakes.

    (b) diamond back and striped snakes.

    (c) pit vipers and cardiotoxic snakes.

    (d) All of the above.

    (e) None of the above.

205. The most dangerous snake bites are from

    (a) neurotoxic snakes.

    (b) cardiotoxic snakes.

    (c) inguinal snakes.

    (d) pit vipers.

    (e) reclusive snakes.

206. Pit vipers have

    (a) black and red bands separated by white or yellow bands, and round pupils.

    (b) triangular heads with a pit below each eye.

    (c) color patterns that vary, and elliptical pupils.

    (d) Both answers (a) and (b).

    (e) Both answers (b) and (c).

207. Coral snakes have

    (a) black and red bands separated by white or yellow bands, and round pupils.

    (b) triangular heads with a pit below each eye.

    (c) color patterns that vary, and elliptical pupils.

    (d) Both answers (a) and (b).

    (e) Both answers (b) and (c).

208. Pit viper bites are noted to present with

    (a) teeth marks only, sometimes in double rows.

    (b) fang marks (may be only one if bite was uneven).

    (c) only minor pain or numbness at the site.

    (d) Both answers (a) and (c).

    (e) Both answers (b) and (c).

209. Coral snake bites are noted to present with

    (a) teeth marks only, sometimes in double rows.
    (b) fang marks (may be only one if bite was uneven).
    (c) only minor pain or numbness at the site.
    (d) Both answers (a) and (c).
    (e) Both answers (b) and (c).

210. Nonpoisonous snake bites are noted to present with

    (a) teeth marks only, sometimes in double rows.
    (b) fang marks (may be only one if bite was uneven).
    (c) only minor pain or numbness at the site.
    (d) Both answers (a) and (c).
    (e) Both answers (b) and (c).

211. Which of the following statements regarding treatment of snake bites is true?

    (a) Apply constricting bands above and below the bite; the blood will carry the toxin to the heart if a pulse can still be felt distal to the lower band.
    (b) Apply ice to all snake bites to slow the spread of the toxin.
    (c) Encourage movement of the bitten extremity to diminish pain and edema.
    (d) Cut open the wound with a sterile scalpel and suction with a cup only if the bite is less than 30 minutes old, the patient shows signs of envenomation, and a physician has ordered you to do so.
    (e) Transport the patient with lights and sirens, even if the vital signs appear stable (the patient may deteriorate suddenly).

212. The primary pacemaker of the heart is located in

    (a) the right ventricle.
    (b) the left ventricle.
    (c) the right atrium.
    (d) the left atrium.
    (e) the brain.

213. The arteries that supply the heart muscle with blood are called the _____ arteries.

    (a) cardiac
    (b) myoepithelium
    (c) myocardium
    (d) coronary
    (e) myocarditis

214. The muscle tissue of the heart is called the _____.

    (a) cardiac

    (b) myoepithelium

    (c) myocardium

    (d) coronary

    (e) myocarditis

215. An accumulation of fatty deposits along the interior walls of the arteries is called

    (a) arteriostenosis.

    (b) an aneurysm.

    (c) atherosclerosis.

    (d) arteriosclerosis.

    (e) arteritis.

216. When there is thickening, hardening, and loss of elasticity of the walls of the arteries, the condition is called

    (a) arteriostenosis.

    (b) an aneurysm.

    (c) atherosclerosis.

    (d) arteriosclerosis.

    (e) arteritis.

217. A weakened area of an artery that begins to stretch and bulge (and may rupture) is called

    (a) arteriostenosis.

    (b) an aneurysm.

    (c) atherosclerosis.

    (d) arteriosclerosis.

    (e) arteritis.

218. Waste products and fat that stick to the interior walls of blood vessels gradually form a substance called

    (a) plasma.

    (b) emboli.

    (c) plaque.

    (d) a thrombus.

    (e) an embolus.

219. A single mass of tissue, fat, clotted blood, or a bubble of air that is loose and traveling through the circulatory system is called

    (a) plasma.

    (b) emboli.

(c) plaque.

(d) a thrombus.

(e) an embolus.

220. Several masses of tissue, fat, clotted blood, or bubbles of air that are loose and traveling through the circulatory system are called

(a) plasma.

(b) emboli.

(c) plaque.

(d) a thrombus.

(e) an embolus.

221. When an area collects excessive amounts of waste or fats so that a bulge is created, diminishing the size of the vessel, that bulge is called

(a) plasma.

(b) emboli.

(c) plaque.

(d) a thrombus.

(e) an embolus.

222. When atherosclerosis or an embolus causes a complete blockage in an artery, the blockage is called an

(a) occlusion.

(b) infarction.

(c) impaction.

(d) infraction.

(e) ossification.

223. When the blockage occurs, the tissue beyond it begins to die, creating an area of dead tissue called an

(a) occlusion.

(b) infarction.

(c) impaction.

(d) infraction.

(e) ossification.

224. When a coronary artery is narrowed but not blocked

(a) the patient has angina pectoris on exertion.

(b) the patient has an acute myocardial infarction beyond the site.

(c) the patient has pulmonary edema.

(d) the patient's heart will immediately stop pumping.

(e) the patient will die despite rescuers' efforts to save him.

225. When a coronary artery becomes totally blocked
  (a) the patient has angina pectoris on exertion.
  (b) the patient has an acute myocardial infarction beyond the site.
  (c) the patient has pulmonary edema.
  (d) the patient's heart will immediately stop pumping.
  (e) the patient will die despite rescuers' efforts to save him.

226. Which of the following statements regarding nitroglycerin (NTG) is false?
  (a) Nitroglycerin comes in tablet and paste forms.
  (b) Nitroglycerin may relieve chest pain by dilating the coronary arteries to provide better oxygenation to the heart muscle.
  (c) Nitroglycerin may cause the patient's blood pressure to increase by dilating the coronary arteries and providing better blood flow to the ventricles.
  (d) Nitroglycerin comes in patches and spray forms.
  (e) Nitroglycerin tablets are not to be swallowed; they are placed under the patient's tongue to dissolve there.

227. Which of the following statements regarding nitroglycerin is true?
  (a) Nitroglycerin is not to be taken more frequently than every 5 minutes.
  (b) No more than 3 nitroglycerin tablets should be taken for a single episode of angina.
  (c) If the conscious patient's systolic blood pressure is less than 90, do not allow him to have even one nitroglycerin tablet.
  (d) All of the above are true.
  (e) None of the above is true.

228. Which of the following statements regarding nitroglycerin is false?
  (a) Nitroglycerin dilates all of the body's arteries and frequently causes a severe headache.
  (b) If 3 nitroglycerin have not relieved the patient's chest pain, the patient is having an acute myocardial infarction.
  (c) Fresh nitroglycerin will normally produce a burning or "tingling" sensation under the tongue.
  (d) All of the above are false.
  (e) None of the above is false.

229. Which of the following statements regarding acute myocardial infarction is true?

 (a) The heart may still continue to pump when a part of the muscle dies.
 (b) The most frequent site of acute myocardial infarction is the left ventricle.
 (c) If too much muscle dies, shock or sudden death will result.
 (d) All of the above are true.
 (e) None of the above is true.

230. Which of the following statements regarding acute myocardial infarction is false?

 (a) Acute myocardial infarction may be accompanied by pulmonary edema without peripheral edema.
 (b) Acute myocardial infarction may occur without chest pain.
 (c) Acute myocardial infarction patients who have any signs or symptoms of shock should receive high-flow oxygen even if they have COPD.
 (d) All of the above are false.
 (e) None of the above is false.

231. Which of the following statements regarding congestive heart failure is true?

 (a) Congestive heart failure may be accompanied by pulmonary edema without peripheral edema.
 (b) Congestive heart failure may occur without chest pain.
 (c) Congestive heart failure patients who have any signs or symptoms of shock should receive high-flow oxygen even if they have COPD.
 (d) All of the above are true.
 (e) None of the above is true.

232. Which of the following statements regarding congestive heart failure is true?

 (a) Left ventricular failure will cause fluids to first accumulate in the patient's ankles.
 (b) Right ventricular failure will cause fluids to first accumulate in the patient's lungs.
 (c) Right ventricular failure will cause distended neck veins.
 (d) All of the above are true.
 (e) None of the above is true.

233. Accumulation of fluids in the lungs is called
  (a) peripheral edema.
  (b) pulmonary edema.
  (c) pedal edema.
  (d) Both answers (a) and (b).
  (e) Both answers (a) and (c).

234. Accumulation of fluids in the feet and ankles is called
  (a) peripheral edema.
  (b) pulmonary edema.
  (c) pedal edema.
  (d) Both answers (a) and (b).
  (e) Both answers (a) and (c).

235. Accumulation of fluids in the fingers and hands is called
  (a) peripheral edema.
  (b) pulmonary edema.
  (c) pedal edema.
  (d) Both answers (a) and (b).
  (e) Both answers (a) and (c).

236. Accumulation of fluids in the abdomen is called
  (a) peripheral edema.
  (b) pulmonary edema.
  (c) rebound.
  (d) ascities.
  (e) dyspnea.

237. Sudden onset of weakness, nausea, and sweating may indicate
  (a) an acute myocardial infarction.
  (b) angina pectoris.
  (c) congestive heart failure.
  (d) Answers (a) and (b) only.
  (e) Answers (a), (b), and (c).

238. Sudden death (without warning signs and symptoms) is caused by
  (a) an acute myocardial infarction.
  (b) angina pectoris.
  (c) congestive heart failure.
  (d) Answers (a) and (c) only.
  (e) Answers (a), (b), and (c).

239. Substernal chest pain with radiation to the jaw, back, and/or arms may indicate
    (a) an acute myocardial infarction.
    (b) angina pectoris.
    (c) congestive heart failure.
    (d) Answers (a) and (b) only.
    (e) Answers (a), (b), and (c).

240. When the heart does not pump blood efficiently to the body, causing fluids to accumulate in the extremities or the lungs, the patient has
    (a) an acute myocardial infarction.
    (b) angina pectoris.
    (c) congestive heart failure.
    (d) Answers (a) and (b) only.
    (e) Answers (a), (b), and (c).

241. An irregular pulse may accompany
    (a) an acute myocardial infarction.
    (b) angina pectoris.
    (c) congestive heart failure.
    (d) Answers (a) and (c) only.
    (e) Answers (a), (b), and (c).

242. Chest pain that wakes a patient from sleep may accompany
    (a) an acute myocardial infarction.
    (b) angina pectoris.
    (c) congestive heart failure.
    (d) Answers (a) and (c) only.
    (e) Answers (a),(b), and (c).

243. A blood pressure that is normal or high may accompany
    (a) an acute myocardial infarction.
    (b) angina pectoris.
    (c) congestive heart failure.
    (d) Answers (a) and (c) only.
    (e) Answers (a), (b), and (c).

244. Chest pain that is relieved by rest may accompany

    (a) an acute myocardial infarction.

    (b) angina pectoris.

    (c) congestive heart failure.

    (d) Answers (a) and (b) only.

    (e) Answers (a), (b), and (c).

245. Hypotension may accompany

    (a) an acute myocardial infarction.

    (b) angina pectoris.

    (c) congestive heart failure.

    (d) Answers (a) and (c) only.

    (e) Answers (a), (b), and (c).

246. Chest pain brought on by exertion or stress can be related to

    (a) an acute myocardial infarction.

    (b) angina pectoris.

    (c) congestive heart failure.

    (d) Answers (a) and (b) only.

    (e) Answers (a), (b), and (c).

247. Which of the following statements regarding emergency care for angina is false?

    (a) The position of comfort for transport is usually semi-reclining or supine.

    (b) If the patient has a normal or high blood pressure and experiences chest pain, assist the patient to place or spray her nitroglycerin under the tongue.

    (c) Do not allow the patient to ambulate.

    (d) All of the above are false.

    (e) None of the above is false.

248. Which of the following statements regarding emergency care for acute myocardial infarction is true?

    (a) The position of comfort for transport is usually semi-reclining or supine.

    (b) If the patient has a normal or high blood pressure and experiences chest pain, assist the patient to place or spray her nitroglycerin under the tongue.

    (c) Do not allow the patient to ambulate.

    (d) All of the above are true.

    (e) None of the above is true.

249. Which of the following statements regarding emergency care for congestive heart failure is false?
- (a) The position of comfort for transport is usually semi-reclining or supine.
- (b) If the patient has a normal or high blood pressure and experiences chest pain, assist the patient to place or spray her nitroglycerin under the tongue.
- (c) Do not allow the patient to ambulate.
- (d) All of the above are false.
- (e) None of the above is false.

250. The medical term for a stroke is
- (a) craniovascular accident (CVA).
- (b) cerebrovascular accident (CVA).
- (c) coronaryvascular accident (CVA).
- (d) All of the above.
- (e) None of the above.

251. A CVA can be caused by all of the following, except
- (a) head trauma.
- (b) a psychiatric disorder.
- (c) a fat embolus from atherosclerosis.
- (d) a blood embolus produced in the heart because of an irregular heart beat.
- (e) the rupture of an artery in the brain.

252. Signs and symptoms of CVA include all of the following, except
- (a) numbness or paralysis of both arms and/or both legs.
- (b) confusion, altered level of conciousness, or unconciousness.
- (c) dizziness, seizures, and/or difficulty with speech or vision.
- (d) headache without other symptoms.
- (e) incontinence of feces and/or urine.

253. Which of the following statements regarding emergency care for a CVA victim is false?

    (a) Care will depend on the signs and symptoms exhibited by the patient.

    (b) The airway must be monitored continuously.

    (c) Even if the patient is unconscious, nasal cannula oxygen at 2 LPM is sufficient.

    (d) Even though the patient may be unable to speak or appears unconscious, she can probably hear everything you are saying.

    (e) Repeated neurological evaluation is an important part of the EMT's responsibilities.

254. Medical causes of difficulty in breathing include all of the following, except

    (a) CVA, AMI, CHF, or pneumonia.

    (b) hyperventilation and psychological stress.

    (c) asthma, allergic reactions, or airway obstruction by aspiration of vomitus.

    (d) chronic obstructive lung diseases.

    (e) an open sucking chest wound.

255. The medical term for difficulty in breathing is

    (a) asphyxia.

    (b) aphasia.

    (c) dyspnea.

    (d) apnea.

    (e) tachpnea.

256. The medical term for inability to coordinate speech (incoherent or slurred speech) is

    (a) asphyxia.

    (b) aphasia.

    (c) dyspnea.

    (d) apnea.

    (e) tachpnea.

257. The medical term for rapid breathing is

    (a) asphyxia.

    (b) aphasia.

    (c) dyspnea.

    (d) apnea.

    (e) tachpnea.

258. The medical term for the absence of respirations is
- (a) asphyxia.
- (b) aphasia.
- (c) dyspnea.
- (d) apnea.
- (e) tachpnea.

259. The medical term for suffocation is
- (a) asphyxia.
- (b) aphasia.
- (c) dyspnea.
- (d) apnea.
- (e) tachpnea.

260. In the patient without COPD, the primary stimulus for breathing is
- (a) a low level of carbon dioxide in the arterial blood.
- (b) a high level of carbon dioxide in the arterial blood.
- (c) a high level of oxygen in the arterial blood.
- (d) a low level of oxygen in the arterial blood.
- (e) an equal level of oxygen and carbon dioxide in the arterial blood.

261. In the patient without COPD, the secondary stimulus for breathing is
- (a) a low level of carbon dioxide in the arterial blood.
- (b) a high level of carbon dioxide in the arterial blood.
- (c) a high level of oxygen in the arterial blood.
- (d) a low level of oxygen in the arterial blood.
- (e) an equal level of oxygen and carbon dioxide in the arterial blood.

262. In the COPD patient, the primary stimulus for breathing is
- (a) a low level of carbon dioxide in the arterial blood.
- (b) a high level of carbon dioxide in the arterial blood.
- (c) a high level of oxygen in the arterial blood.
- (d) a low level of oxygen in the arterial blood.
- (e) an equal level of oxygen and carbon dioxide in the arterial blood.

263. The patient with _____ typically appears cyanotic, has extremity edema, and a productive cough.
- (a) asthma
- (b) chronic bronchitis
- (c) emphysema
- (d) All of the above.
- (e) None of the above.

264. The patient with _____ typically appears pale or pink, has a barrel-shaped chest, and breathes in small puffs against pursed lips.
- (a) asthma
- (b) chronic bronchitis
- (c) emphysema
- (d) All of the above.
- (e) None of the above.

265. The patient with _____ typically appears and functions normally in between attacks of shortness of breath.
- (a) asthma
- (b) chronic bronchitis
- (c) emphysema
- (d) All of the above.
- (e) None of the above.

266. *Hypoxic drive* can be defined as
- (a) a change in the primary breathing stimulus, so that the patient's respiratory drive is primarily triggered by low oxygen levels in the arterial blood.
- (b) the term that applies to the primary breathing stimulus for COPD patients.
- (c) a breathing stimulus mechanism that produces respiratory arrest in patients unaccustomed to high levels of arterial oxygen.
- (d) All of the above.
- (e) None of the above.

267. Which of the following statements regarding treatment for the patient with emphysema is true?
- (a) Supplemental oxygen should be delivered by nasal cannula or venturi mask.
- (b) If the patient has serious medical complaints in addition to his respiratory disease, administer high-flow oxygen.
- (c) Administer high-flow oxygen and assist the patient in using her inhaler of medication according to directions

on the label.
  (d) Both answers (a) and (b) are true.
  (e) Answers (a), (b), and (c) are true.

268. Which of the following statements regarding treatment for the patient with chronic bronchitis is true?
  (a) Supplemental oxygen should be delivered by nasal cannula or venturi mask.
  (b) If the patient has serious medical complaints in addition to his respiratory disease, administer high-flow oxygen.
  (c) Administer high-flow oxygen and assist the patient in using her inhaler of medication according to directions on the label.
  (d) Both answers (a) and (b) are true.
  (e) Answers (a), (b), and (c) are true.

269. Which of the following statements regarding treatment for the patient with asthma is true?
  (a) Supplemental oxygen should be delivered by nasal cannula or venturi mask.
  (b) If the patient has serious medical complaints in addition to his respiratory disease, administer high-flow oxygen.
  (c) Administer high-flow oxygen and assist the patient in using her inhaler of medication according to directions on the label.
  (d) Both answers (a) and (b) are true.
  (e) Answers (a), (b), and (c) are true.

270. Which of the following statements regarding hyperventilation is false?
  (a) Hyperventilation is almost always due to psychological stress.
  (b) Hyperventilation frequently causes numbness, tingling, and/or spasms of the hands and fingers, and the feet and toes.
  (c) Hyperventilation frequently causes numbness or tingling around the mouth.
  (d) Psychogenic hyperventilation rarely causes cyanosis.
  (e) Hyperventilation can be a sign of severe head injury, hypoxia, acute myocardial infarction, stroke, or other serious medical conditions.

271. All of the following signs and symptoms are shared by acute myocardial infarction and hyperventilation, except

    (a) anxiety, dizziness, and fainting.

    (b) tachypnea.

    (c) numbness or tingling of the arms and/or hands.

    (d) pulmonary edema.

    (e) stabbing chest pain.

272. Which of the following statements regarding spontaneous pneumothorax is false?

    (a) In the absence of trauma, a patient will not develop a tension pneumothorax.

    (b) A congenital anomaly within the lungs may result in a spontaneous pneumothorax.

    (c) Lung cancer may cause a spontaneous pneumothorax.

    (d) Scar tissue from previous surgeries or old injuries may rupture or leak, causing a spontaneous pneumothorax.

    (e) All of the signs and symptoms produced by traumatic pneumothorax may be exhibited by the patient with a spontaneous pneumothorax.

The answer key for Test Section Two is on page 217.

Test
Section
Three

Test Section Three covers the following subjects and their treatment:

* Diabetes
* Acute Abdomen
* Communicable Diseases
* Substance Abuse
* Pediatric Patients
* Bleeding and Shock
* Vital Signs
* Anti-shock Garments (PASG or MAST)
* Soft Tissue Injuries
* Fractures and Dislocations of the Upper and Lower Extremities
* Heat Injuries
* Hypothermia and Frostbite
* Water-related Injuries
* Medical Terminology

EMT - Basic
National Standards Review Self Test

1.   Abdominal distress caused by irritation or inflammation of the peritoneum is called
     (a) rebound sign.
     (b) acute melena.
     (c) acute gastritis.
     (d) acute abdomen.
     (e) acute diverticulitis.

2.   Which of the following statements regarding diabetes is false?
     (a) Diabetes is a condition in which the body is unable to produce enough insulin to use sugar normally.
     (b) Body cells cannot survive without sugar.
     (c) Insulin enables sugar to pass from the body cells to the blood stream for excretion.
     (d) If there is not enough insulin, sugar will be unable to get into the body cells and they will starve.
     (e) If there is too much insulin, brain cells will begin to die from lack of sugar in the blood.

3.   Insulin shock is another name for
     (a) hyperglycemia.
     (b) hypoglycemia.
     (c) alcohol intoxication.
     (d) Either answer (a) or (b).
     (e) None of the above.

4.   Diabetic coma is another name for
     (a) hyperglycemia.
     (b) hypoglycemia.
     (c) alcohol intoxication.
     (d) Either answer (a) or (b).
     (e) None of the above.

5.   When an excessive amount of insulin causes insufficient availability of sugar for the brain cells, the patient is suffering from
     (a) hyperglycemia.
     (b) hypoglycemia.

    (c) alcohol intoxication.

    (d) Either answer (a) or (b).

    (e) None of the above.

6.   A diabetic patient who doesn't follow his doctor's orders regarding food and insulin intake may suffer

    (a) hyperglycemia.

    (b) hypoglycemia.

    (c) alcohol intoxication.

    (d) Either answer (a) or (b).

    (e) None of the above.

7.   When there is insufficient insulin available, the body cells are not able to take in sugar and the patient will suffer from

    (a) hyperglycemia.

    (b) hypoglycemia.

    (c) alcohol intoxication.

    (d) Either answer (a) or (b).

    (e) None of the above.

8.   The onset of _____ is gradual; over a period of days.

    (a) hyperglycemia

    (b) hypoglycemia

    (c) alcohol intoxication

    (d) Either answer (a) or (b).

    (e) None of the above.

9.   The onset of _____ is rapid; it may occur within minutes.

    (a) hyperglycemia

    (b) hypoglycemia

    (c) alcohol intoxication

    (d) Either answer (a) or (b).

    (e) None of the above.

10.   Pale, moist skin and a full, rapid pulse may indicate

    (a) hyperglycemia.

    (b) hypoglycemia.

    (c) alcohol intoxication.

    (d) Either answer (a) or (b).

    (e) None of the above.

11.   Your patient's breath smells of alcohol; she is dishevelled and filthy. The bartender says that she's a regular customer and a heavy drinker, but now is acting very abnormally. Your patient may be suffering from

(a) hyperglycemia.
(b) hypoglycemia.
(c) alcohol intoxication.
(d) Either answer (a) or (b).
(e) None of the above.

12.   Dry, warm skin with a rapid, weak pulse may indicate

(a) hyperglycemia.
(b) hypoglycemia.
(c) alcohol intoxication.
(d) Either answer (a) or (b).
(e) None of the above.

13.   _____ causes the patient to have rapid, deep respirations with sweet or fruity-smelling breath.

(a) Hyperglycemia
(b) Hypoglycemia
(c) Alcohol intoxication
(d) Either answer (a) or (b).
(e) None of the above.

14.   Seizures may be caused by

(a) hyperglycemia.
(b) hypoglycemia.
(c) alcohol intoxication.
(d) Either answer (a) or (b).
(e) All of the above.

15.   Combativeness and disorientation may indicate

(a) hyperglycemia.
(b) hypoglycemia.
(c) alcohol intoxication.
(d) Either answer (a) or (b).
(e) None of the above.

16.   Recently excessive urination with increased thirst and fluid intake may indicate that a diabetic is

(a) hyperglycemic.
(b) normoglycemic.

(c) hypoglycemic.

(d) anemic.

(e) Either answer (a) or (b).

17. A diabetic may become _____ if he has recently had nausea and vomiting from a minor illness.

(a) hyperglycemic.

(b) normoglycemic.

(c) hypoglycemic.

(d) anemic.

(e) Either answer (a) or (b).

18. Excessive exercise or overexertion can cause a diabetic to become

(a) hyperglycemic.

(b) normoglycemic.

(c) hypoglycemic.

(d) anemic.

(e) Either answer (a) or (b).

19. Overeating or forgetting to take his insulin may cause a diabetic to become

(a) hyperglycemic.

(b) normoglycemic.

(c) hypoglycemic.

(d) anemic.

(e) Either answer (a) or (b).

20. Which of the following statements regarding treatment of diabetic emergencies is false?

(a) Any form of sugar can be given to a conscious patient.

(b) Do not administer any form of oral sugar to an unconscious patient.

(c) Brain damage or death may occur if a patient remains hypoglycemic.

(d) Do not administer sugar in any form to a patient you believe to be hyperglycemic.

(e) Both the hyperglycemic and hypoglycemic patient need oxygen and transportation to a medical facility.

21.   A violent involuntary contraction or series of contractions of the skeletal muscles is called

    (a) a seizure.
    (b) a convulsion.
    (c) status epilepticus.
    (d) an epileptic fit.
    (e) status convulsiveness.

22.   A sudden attack of epilepsy is called

    (a) a seizure.
    (b) a convulsion.
    (c) status epilepticus.
    (d) an epileptic fit.
    (e) status convulsiveness.

23.   Repeated attacks of involuntary skeletal muscle contractions without regaining consciousness between them is called

    (a) a seizure.
    (b) a convulsion.
    (c) status epilepticus.
    (d) an epileptic fit.
    (e) status convulsiveness.

24.   Causes of epilepsy, seizures, or convulsions include all of the following, except

    (a) fever, infections, or diseases.
    (b) head injury or hypoxia.
    (c) alcohol or drug abuse.
    (d) cervical spine injury.
    (e) pregnancy.

25.   During _____ the patient has convulsions or an altered level of consciousness due to abnormal stimulation of brain cells.

    (a) an epileptic fit
    (b) a grand mal seizure
    (c) a petit mal seizure
    (d) Either answer (a) or (b).
    (e) Either answer (b) or (c).

26. During _____ there are tonic and clonic convulsions, and the patient may be incontinent of urine and/or feces.
    (a) an epileptic fit
    (b) a grand mal seizure
    (c) a petit mal seizure
    (d) Either answer (a) or (b).
    (e) Either answer (b) or (c).

27. During _____ the patient always loses consciousness.
    (a) an epileptic fit
    (b) a grand mal seizure
    (c) a petit mal seizure
    (d) Either answer (a) or (b).
    (e) Either answer (b) or (c).

28. After _____ has occured, the patient may experience a period of confusion or fatigue, called a *postictal state*.
    (a) an epileptic fit
    (b) a grand mal seizure
    (c) a petit mal seizure
    (d) Either answer (a) or (b).
    (e) Either answer (b) or (c).

29. Which of the following statements regarding emergency treatment of seizures is true?
    (a) During a grand mal seizure, the patient will require physical restraints to prevent head or extremity injuries.
    (b) It is important to gently force a bite block between the patient's teeth to prevent dental injuries or self-inflicted bites.
    (c) After the seizure, it is important to pull the tongue forward with a gloved hand, to prevent the patient from swallowing his tongue.
    (d) All of the above are true.
    (e) None of the above is true.

30. Common causes of acute abdominal distress include all of the following, except
    (a) peritonitis, pancreatitis, or hepatitis.
    (b) an ectopic pregnancy.
    (c) meningitis.
    (d) a gallstone or kidney stone.
    (e) an abdominal aortic aneurysm.

31. Acute abdominal distress may exhibit any of the following signs and symptoms, except

  (a) hypotension.
  (b) normal or elevated blood pressure (in the presence of extreme pain).
  (c) localized abdominal pain.
  (d) diffuse abdominal pain.
  (e) rapid, shallow breathing with a slow pulse.

32. Acute abdominal distress may exhibit any of the following signs and symptoms, except

  (a) refusal to allow palpation of the abdomen.
  (b) the patient lies as still as possible and is reluctant to move despite the degree of pain and restlessness.
  (c) tense, often distended abdomen with or without nausea and vomiting.
  (d) the patient prefers to lie supine with outstretched legs.
  (e) complaints of recent constipation or diarrhea.

33. Universal precautions utilized by health care providers to protect against communicable diseases include all of the following, except

  (a) plastic goggles.
  (b) soap and water washing of hands and face.
  (c) avoiding direct contact with the patient's body.
  (d) use of disposable latex gloves.
  (e) wearing of disposable gowns and masks.

34. A patient sneezing or coughing into your face may result in _____ transmission of disease.

  (a) direct contact
  (b) indirect contact
  (c) airborne droplet contact
  (d) All of the above.
  (e) None of the above.

35. Touching the patient's infected blood, feces, urine, mucous, saliva, or perspiration may result in _____ transmission of disease.

  (a) direct contact
  (b) indirect contact
  (c) airborne droplet contact
  (d) All of the above.
  (e) None of the above.

36. Handling contaminated linen, clothing, or garbage may result in _____ transmission of disease.
    (a) direct contact
    (b) indirect contact
    (c) airborne droplet contact
    (d) All of the above.
    (e) None of the above.

37. Alcohol
    (a) is a central nervous system depressant.
    (b) is a central nervous system stimulant.
    (c) is a sedative.
    (d) causes a psychological disease only.
    (e) causes a physical disease only.

38. Which of the following signs and symptoms of alcohol intoxication are also possible indications of a medical emergency?
    (a) Swaying, unsteadiness, and slurred speech.
    (b) Nausea, vomiting, and incontinence of feces or urine.
    (c) Sweet, fruity odor on the breath.
    (d) All of the above.
    (e) None of the above.

39. Which of the following statements regarding alcohol intoxication is false?
    (a) Alcohol can cause death by paralyzing the respiratory center of the brain.
    (b) The acetone breath odor of a diabetic is clearly distinguishable from the odor of alcohol on the breath.
    (c) Tranquilizers, barbiturates, or antihistimines taken in combination with alcohol may produce depressant effects far greater than that of the medication.
    (d) All of the above are false.
    (e) None of the above is false.

40. The EMT's primary concerns, when treating a patient whose illness or injury is compounded by alcohol or drug intoxication, includes all of the following, except

(a) anticipation of combativeness and routine application of soft restraints.

(b) anticipation of hidden injuries with liberal use of spinal immobilization.

(c) anticipation of respiratory depression or arrest.

(d) anticipation of allergic reactions and shock.

(e) anticipation of vomiting and potential aspiration.

41. The term "DTs" is used to indicate

(a) delirious tremors.

(b) diabetic tremors.

(c) diverse tremors.

(d) deadly tremens.

(e) delirium tremens.

42. An alcoholic may suffer alcohol withdrawal or DTs because

(a) illness, injury, or lack of funds has prevented her from obtaining as much alcohol as her system is accustomed to consume.

(b) her blood-alcohol level has dropped below her normal level.

(c) she has quit drinking.

(d) All of the above.

(e) None of the above.

43. Signs and symptoms of alcohol withdrawal include all of the following, except

(a) seizures.

(b) extremity tremors, restlessness, or confusion.

(c) euphoria, elation, or excessive laughing and joking.

(d) hallucinations or delusions.

(e) combative or suicidal behavior.

44. Which of the following statements regarding amphetamine abuse is false?

(a) Blood pressure, breathing, and general body activity are decreased.

(b) Respiratory failure can occur with cocaine use.

(c) After a run of repeated high doses, the user is exhausted and sleeps. When he wakes, he experiences elation or euphoria, and is eager for another "fix."

(d) All of the above are false.

(e) None of the above is false.

45. Barbiturates, opiates, and tranquilizers are
(a) central nervous system stimulants ("uppers").
(b) central nervous system depressants ("downers").
(c) hallucinogens ("psychedelics").
(d) All of the above.
(e) None of the above.

46. LSD, mescaline, and psilocybin are
(a) central nervous system stimulants ("uppers").
(b) central nervous system depressants ("downers").
(c) hallucinogens ("psychedelics").
(d) All of the above.
(e) None of the above.

47. Cocaine and caffeine are
(a) central nervous system stimulants ("uppers").
(b) central nervous system depressants ("downers").
(c) hallucinogens ("psychedelics").
(d) All of the above.
(e) None of the above.

48. Which of the following statements regarding barbiturate abuse is true?
(a) Barbiturates include Nembutal, Seconal, and phenobarbital.
(b) Barbiturate overdose can produce respiratory depression, unconsciousness, and death.
(c) Withdrawal from barbiturates can cause anxiety, tremors, nausea, fever, delirium, seizures, or death.
(d) All of the above are true.
(e) None of the above is true.

49. Which of the following statements regarding tranquilizer abuse is false?
(a) Tranquilizers include Miltown, Equanil, and Valium.
(b) Tranquilizer overdose can produce respiratory depression, unconsciousness, and death.
(c) Withdrawal from tranquilizers can cause anxiety, tremors, nausea, fever, delirium, seizures, or death.
(d) All of the above are false.
(e) None of the above is false.

50. Which of the following statements regarding opiates (narcotics) is false?

    (a) Opiates include Benzedrine, Dexedrine, and cocaine.

    (b) Narcotics are used medicinally to relieve pain and anxiety.

    (c) Overdose of opiates can result in deep sleep, unconsciousness, respiratory depression, and death.

    (d) The pupils of opiate users are described as "pinpoint" in size.

    (e) Withdrawal from narcotics causes intense agitation, abdominal discomfort, dilated pupils, increased respiratory rate, fever, and a strong craving for a "fix."

51. A person who inhales paint, glue, or other solvents (gasoline, lighter fluid, nail polish, and the like) can

    (a) experience effects similar to those of alcohol.

    (b) die because of suffocation.

    (c) die because of changes in the rhythm of the heartbeat.

    (d) All of the above.

    (e) None of the above.

52. Which of the following statements regarding hallucinogen abuse is false?

    (a) These drugs include morning glory seeds and peyote.

    (b) They produce changes in mood and sensory awareness.

    (c) The user may proclaim she can "hear" colors or "see" sounds.

    (d) Acute cases of a "bad trip" need medical attention.

    (e) Hallucinogens produce elation and euphoria, causing the user to present a danger to himself, but not a danger to others.

53. Medically speaking, the age range of an infant is defined as

    (a) less than 6 months old.

    (b) less than 1 year old.

    (c) 6 months to 18 years old.

    (d) 1 to 18 years old.

    (e) less than 18 years old.

54. Medically speaking, the age range of a child is defined as

    (a) less than 6 months old.

    (b) less than 1 year old.

    (c) 6 months to 18 years old.

(d) 1 to 18 years old.

(e) less than 18 years old.

55. Which of the following statements regarding pediatric trauma is false?

(a) Little blood loss is required for the infant or small child to go into shock.

(b) A child who appears drowsy, disinterested, or fatigued may be suffering from a head injury.

(c) Children frequently suffer first- and second-degree burns to the face and hands.

(d) A "bike fork compression injury" is a crushing injury of the wrist.

(e) A 12-month-old child with a pulse of 120 is not tachycardic.

56. Which of the following statements regarding child abuse is false?

(a) An infant or small child may die as a result of being vigorously shaken to "shut him up!"

(b) Child abuse is frequently quite obvious and must be reported to the authorities.

(c) Psychological injury is a form of child abuse.

(d) Failure to provide appropriate nutrition, hygiene, clothing, shelter, or safety is a form of child abuse called *neglect.*

(e) If you suspect child abuse, do not ask the child about it, but report your suspicions to the emergency room staff.

57. Which of the following statements regarding pediatric sexual assault is true?

(a) Any injury to a child's genitals is an indication of sexual assault.

(b) You should kindly but firmly insist that the child tell you how the injury occurred.

(c) Do not question a child about sexual abuse unless the parents or guardians are present.

(d) Do not document suspicions of abuse or assault, but verbally report them to the emergency room staff.

(e) Since the advent of television programs concerning sexual abuse, children will frequently lie about sexual assault in order to punish an adult who has angered them.

58.   Which of the following statements regarding pediatric patients with fevers is true?

(a)   Fever rarely accompanies life-threatening illness.

(b)   If a fever becomes too severe, the child will have a febrile seizure to reduce the body temperature, and there will no longer be a need for medical treatment.

(c)   Only those fevers accompanied by stiffness in the neck or back are considered significant emergencies.

(d)   All of the above are true.

(e)   None of the above is true.

59.   Respiratory distress with fever, drooling, fear of swallowing, and resistance to lying down indicates a child suffering from

(a)   croup.

(b)   epiglottitis.

(c)   whooping cough.

(d)   Both answers (a) and (b).

(e)   Both answers (a) and (c).

60.   Respiratory distress with fever and a loud, barklike cough indicates a child suffering from

(a)   croup.

(b)   epiglottitis.

(c)   whooping cough.

(d)   Both answers (a) and (b).

(e)   Both answers (a) and (c).

61.   High-flow, humidified oxygen should be administered to any child suffering from

(a)   croup.

(b)   epiglottitis.

(c)   whooping cough.

(d)   Both answers (a) and (b).

(e)   Both answers (a) and (c).

62.   A conscious child should never be placed supine if suffering from

(a)   croup.

(b)   epiglottitis.

(c)   whooping cough.

(d)   Both answers (a) and (b).

(e)   Both answers (a) and (c).

63.   An oral airway should never be used if the child is unconscious and the suspected cause is

   (a) croup.
   (b) epiglottitis.
   (c) whooping cough.
   (d) Both answers (a) and (b).
   (e) Both answers (a) and (c).

64.   Respiratory distress with coughing and wheezing, but without fever, indicates a child suffering from

   (a) bronchitis.
   (b) bronchiolitis.
   (c) asthma.
   (d) Answers (a) and (b) only.
   (e) Any of the above.

65.   Pediatric _____ may precede anaphlactic shock.

   (a) bronchitis
   (b) bronchiolitis
   (c) asthma
   (d) Both answers (a) and (b).
   (e) Any of the above.

66.   High-flow, humidified oxygen should be administered to any
child suffering from

   (a) bronchitis.
   (b) bronchiolitis.
   (c) asthma.
   (d) Both answers (a) and (b).
   (e) Any of the above.

67.   Which of the following statements regarding pediatric poisonings is true?

   (a) An infant or child who overdoses on vitamins may
experience nausea, vomiting, unconsciousness, and
death.
   (b) Small children are the most common victims of
poisoning.
   (c) Aspirin, petroleum product, or lead poisonings are life-
threatening in the pediatric patient.
   (d) All of the above are true.
   (e) None of the above is true.

68. Which of the following statements regarding Sudden Infant Death Syndrome (SIDS) is false?

    (a) Child abuse is one of the causes of SIDS.

    (b) Death usually occurs during sleep and SIDS is the leading cause of death in infants less that one year old.

    (c) SIDS occurs in apparently healthy babies without any signs of recent trauma.

    (d) Experts have not determined the cause of SIDS.

    (e) SIDS has been related to periods of apnea during sleep.

69. Leukocytes are

    (a) the watery, fluid portion of the blood.

    (b) responsible for the clotting function of the blood.

    (c) the infection-carrying element of the blood.

    (d) the oxygen-carrying element of the blood.

    (e) the infection-fighting element of the blood.

70. Red blood cells (RBCs) are

    (a) the watery, fluid portion of the blood.

    (b) responsible for the clotting function of the blood.

    (c) the infection-carrying element of the blood.

    (d) the oxygen-carrying element of the blood.

    (e) the infection-fighting element of the blood.

71. White blood cells (WBCs) are

    (a) the watery, fluid portion of the blood.

    (b) responsible for the clotting function of the blood.

    (c) the infection-carrying element of the blood.

    (d) the oxygen-carrying element of the blood.

    (e) the infection-fighting element of the blood.

72. Platelets are

    (a) the watery, fluid portion of the blood.

    (b) responsible for the clotting function of the blood.

    (c) the infection-carrying element of the blood.

    (d) the oxygen-carrying element of the blood.

    (e) the infection-fighting element of the blood.

73. Erythrocytes are

    (a) the watery, fluid portion of the blood.

    (b) responsible for the clotting function of the blood.

    (c) the infection-carrying element of the blood.

    (d) the oxygen-carrying element of the blood.

    (e) the infection-fighting element of the blood.

74. Plasma is
    (a) the watery, fluid portion of the blood.
    (b) responsible for the clotting function of the blood.
    (c) the infection-carrying element of the blood.
    (d) the oxygen-carrying element of the blood.
    (e) the infection-fighting element of the blood.

75. The average adult circulatory system contains approximately _____ liters of blood.
    (a) 4
    (b) 6
    (c) 8
    (d) 10
    (e) 11

76. In the average adult, serious shock will begin soon after the loss of _____ of blood.
    (a) ¼ liter (250 ml)
    (b) ½ liter (500 ml)
    (c) 1 liter (1000 ml)
    (d) 2 liters (2000 ml)
    (e) 3 liters (3000 ml)

77. In the average child, serious shock will begin soon after the loss of _____ of blood.
    (a) ¼ liter (250 ml)
    (b) ½ liter (500 ml)
    (c) 1 liter (1000 ml)
    (d) 2 liters (2000 ml)
    (e) 3 liters (3000 ml)

78. An artery
    (a) carries freshly oxygenated blood to the body.
    (b) is a very thin-walled vessel where exchange of gases, nutrients, and wastes occurs.
    (c) collects deoxygenated blood from the body and carries it back to the heart.
    (d) carries oxygenated blood from the lungs to the heart.
    (e) carries deoxygenated blood from the heart to the lungs.

79.   A vein
  (a) carries freshly oxygenated blood to the body.
  (b) is a very thin-walled vessel where exchange of gases, nutrients, and wastes occurs.
  (c) collects deoxygenated blood from the body and carries it back to the heart.
  (d) carries oxygenated blood from the lungs to the heart.
  (e) carries deoxygenated blood from the heart to the lungs.

80.   A capillary
  (a) carries freshly oxygenated blood to the body.
  (b) is a very thin-walled vessel where exchange of gases, nutrients, and wastes occurs.
  (c) collects deoxygenated blood from the body and carries it back to the heart.
  (d) carries oxygenated blood from the lungs to the heart.
  (e) carries deoxygenated blood from the heart to the lungs.

81.   The pulmonary artery
  (a) carries freshly oxygenated blood to the body.
  (b) is a very thin-walled vessel where exchange of gases, nutrients, and wastes occurs.
  (c) collects deoxygenated blood from the body and carries it back to the heart.
  (d) carries oxygenated blood from the lungs to the heart.
  (e) carries deoxygenated blood from the heart to the lungs.

82.   The pulmonary vein
  (a) carries freshly oxygenated blood to the body.
  (b) is a very thin-walled vessel where exchange of gases, nutrients, and wastes occurs.
  (c) collects deoxygenated blood from the body and carries it back to the heart.
  (d) carries oxygenated blood from the lungs to the heart.
  (e) carries deoxygenated blood from the heart to the lungs.

83.   The term *perfusion* refers to
  (a) the circulation of blood within an organ or body part.
  (b) the exchange of oxygen for carbon dioxide at the capillary level in the body.
  (c) the exchange of nutrients for waste products at the capillary level in the body.
  (d) All of the above.
  (e) None of the above.

84. Bleeding from _____ spurts and is bright red in color.

   (a) a vein
   (b) an artery
   (c) capillaries
   (d) All of the above.
   (e) None of the above.

85. Bleeding from _____ is steady and is dark red in color.

   (a) a vein
   (b) an artery
   (c) capillaries
   (d) All of the above.
   (e) None of the above.

86. Blood oozes from _____ and is dark red in color.

   (a) a vein
   (b) an artery
   (c) capillaries
   (d) All of the above.
   (e) None of the above.

87. Which of the following statements regarding control of bleeding with direct pressure is false?

   (a) Direct pressure will stop most bleeding.
   (b) The pressure dressing should be held in place with a bandage because tape may peel off of moist skin.
   (c) If a dressing becomes saturated with blood, gently replace it with a fresh one, but save the saturated dressings for blood loss estimate in the emergency room.
   (d) All of the above are false.
   (e) None of the above is false.

88. Which of the following statements regarding elevation and pressure points is true?

   (a) Do not elevate an extremity with an impaled object or joint fracture.
   (b) The femoral artery is pressed against the humerus to stop bleeding from the forearm.
   (c) The brachial artery is pressed against the pelvis to stop bleeding in the thigh.
   (d) All of the above are true.
   (e) None of the above is true.

89. Which of the following statements regarding tourniquets is true?

(a) Tourniquets can damage nerves and blood vessels and result in the loss of an arm or leg.

(b) In an emergency, a tourniquet may be temporarily placed and then later removed when there is time to dress the wound appropriately.

(c) All amputations will require a tourniquet.

(d) If the bleeding stops prior to loss of the distal pulse, you must still continue tightening of the tourniquet to prevent internal (hidden) bleeding.

(e) None of the above is true.

90. Which of the following statements regarding hidden, internal bleeding is false?

(a) Internal bleeding can result in severe blood loss and the patient may die of shock.

(b) A closed, fractured femur can result in an internal blood loss of 1000 ml of blood.

(c) Laceration of the liver can result in severe blood loss and quickly be fatal, even in the absence of any other injuries.

(d) All of the above are false.

(e) None of the above is false.

91. Signs and symptoms of serious internal bleeding include all of the following, except

(a) vomiting bright red blood, or dark, "coffee ground" blood.

(b) melena.

(c) pedal edema.

(d) bright red blood in the patient's stool.

(e) hypovolemic shock without external blood loss.

92. Which of the following statements regarding emergency care for internal bleeding is false?

(a) Apply ice packs at the armpits and groin to minimize the flow of blood to the extremities, increasing blood flow to the heart and brain.

(b) Transport using lights and sirens to a trauma center.

(c) A high percentage of oxygen should be administered.

(d) PASG or MAST may be helpful to splint and control internal hemorrhage of the lower extremities.

(e) PASG or MAST may be helpful to control internal abdominal bleeding.

93. Epistaxis may be caused by all of the following, except

   (a) fractured skull or facial bones.

   (b) sinusitis, infections, or abnormalities within the nose.

   (c) bleeding diseases or drug abuse.

   (d) All of the above.

   (e) None of the above.

94. *Shock* is defined as

   (a) the failure of cellular perfusion.

   (b) the period of time following an accident or illness when the patient is hypotensive.

   (c) an extreme psychological reaction to an accident or illness that may produce coma or death.

   (d) All of the above.

   (e) None of the above.

95. Shock is caused by

   (a) failure of the heart to pump blood efficiently.

   (b) severe blood or fluid loss, resulting in insufficient fluid traveling through the circulatory system.

   (c) enlargement of blood vessels so that there is insufficient fluid to fill them.

   (d) breathing problems resulting in inadequate amounts of oxygen available to the body's cells.

   (e) Any of the above causes by itself, or in combination with any of the others.

96. Nausea, vomiting, diarrhea, and excessive urination may cause

   (a) septic shock.

   (b) hypovolemic shock.

   (c) anaphylactic shock.

   (d) metabolic shock.

   (e) psychogenic shock.

97. Severe infections produce bacteria and toxins that cause blood vessels to dilate and leak fluid, resulting in

   (a) septic shock.

   (b) hypovolemic shock.

   (c) anaphylactic shock.

   (d) metabolic shock.

   (e) psychogenic shock.

98. A condition that is considered to be a "self-correcting" form of shock is called

    (a) septic shock.
    (b) hypovolemic shock.
    (c) anaphylactic shock.
    (d) metabolic shock.
    (e) psychogenic shock.

99. A systemic reaction to a bee sting is called

    (a) septic shock.
    (b) hypovolemic shock.
    (c) anaphylactic shock.
    (d) metabolic shock.
    (e) psychogenic shock.

100. Hidden, internal bleeding can produce

    (a) septic shock.
    (b) hypovolemic shock.
    (c) anaphylactic shock.
    (d) metabolic shock.
    (e) psychogenic shock.

101. Syncope, caused by temporary dilation of the blood vessels, resulting in a transiently decreased blood supply to the brain is called

    (a) hemorrhagic shock.
    (b) respiratory shock.
    (c) neurogenic shock.
    (d) psychogenic shock.
    (e) cardiogenic shock.

102. When the heart muscle no longer imparts sufficient contraction to effectively move blood through the circulatory system, it is called

    (a) hemorrhagic shock.
    (b) respiratory shock.
    (c) neurogenic shock.
    (d) psychogenic shock.
    (e) cardiogenic shock.

103. Damage to the spinal cord can cause

    (a) hemorrhagic shock.
    (b) respiratory shock.
    (c) neurogenic shock.

(d) psychogenic shock.
(e) cardiogenic shock.

104. Pulmonary edema results in

(a) hemorrhagic shock.
(b) respiratory shock.
(c) neurogenic shock.
(d) psychogenic shock.
(e) cardiogenic shock.

105. A prolonged and severe epistaxis may result in

(a) hemorrhagic shock.
(b) respiratory shock.
(c) neurogenic shock.
(d) psychogenic shock.
(e) cardiogenic shock.

106. Electrocution will produce

(a) hemorrhagic shock.
(b) respiratory shock.
(c) neurogenic shock.
(d) psychogenic shock.
(e) cardiogenic shock.

107. Which of the following represents the earliest symptom(s) of shock?

(a) Hypotension.
(b) Restlessness, anxiety, and tachycardia.
(c) Nausea, weakness, and thirst.
(d) Cold, pale, and moist skin.
(e) Loss of consciousness.

108. Which of the following represents the earliest sign(s) of shock?

(a) Hypotension.
(b) Restlessness, anxiety, and tachycardia.
(c) Nausea, weakness, and thirst.
(d) Cold, pale, and moist skin.
(e) Loss of consciousness.

109. Which of the following represents the latest sign(s) of shock?

  (a) Hypotension.
  (b) Restlessness, anxiety, and tachycardia.
  (c) Nausea, weakness, and thirst.
  (d) Cold, pale, and moist skin.
  (e) Profound diaphoresis.

110. Capillary refill is considered delayed when a blanched area takes longer than _____ to regain normal color.

  (a) 2 minutes
  (b) 2 seconds
  (c) 1 minute
  (d) 1 second
  (e) 5 seconds

111. *Diaphoresis* is defined as

  (a) pale, cyanotic, or mottled skin.
  (b) a weak and thready pulse.
  (c) profuse sweating.
  (d) marked thirst.
  (e) nausea with vomiting.

112. Which of the following statements regarding the treatment of shock is true?

  (a) Each different form of shock requires different care.
  (b) The basic treatment for shock is to care for the whole patient in an effort to prevent shock from occurring.
  (c) Always provide nasal cannula oxygen to the patient in shock.
  (d) Always keep the shock patient supine to prevent brain death.
  (e) Allow only small sips of water (or small chips of ice) to the shock patient.

113. Treatment of shock includes all of the following, except

  (a) airway management and bleeding control.
  (b) elevation of the lower extremities (unless injuries would be aggravated by doing so).
  (c) splinting of fractures and gentle handling.
  (d) ice packs to reduce internal body temperature and slow the patient's metabolism (to reduce internal bleeding)
  (e) application of MAST or PASG.

114. Which of the following statements regarding anaphylactic shock is false?

(a) Anaphylactic shock may begin as a local allergic reaction to a bite, sting, or plant contact.

(b) Anaphylactic shock develops slowly, usually requiring an hour or more to produce signs and symptoms.

(c) The foreign substance that causes an allergic or anaphylactic reaction is called an *allergen*.

(d) The systemic reaction to the allergen by the body's antibodies causes a histamine release in the circulatory system.

(e) Histamines cause rapid dilation of the blood vessels, and produce hypotension, pulmonary edema, airway spasms, and hives.

115. Allergic reactions and anaphylactic shock can be caused by

(a) insect stings, bites, or other injected substances (including medications).

(b) ingested or inhaled substances.

(c) absorbed substances such as chemicals, skin products, laundry products, or plant contact.

(d) All of the above.

(e) None of the above.

116. All of the following statements represent signs or symptoms of anaphylactic shock, except

(a) the skin may burn, flush, itch, or break out in a rash.

(b) the face and tongue may swell; cyanosis may be visible around the lips.

(c) breathing becomes more and more difficult, and there may be tightness or pain in the chest.

(d) the pulse becomes weaker, and the patient becomes more and more hypertensive.

(e) dizziness and loss of consciousness may ensue, followed rapidly by death.

117. Treatment for anaphylactic shock includes

(a) high-flow oxygen via a nonrebreather mask.

(b) lights and sirens transport to the emergency room.

(c) assisting the patient to inject herself with her epinephrine kit.

(d) Answers (a) and (b) only.

(e) Answers (a), (b), and (c).

118. Which of the following statements regarding pneumatic anti-shock garments (PASG) is false?

(a) PASG may translocate blood from the abdomen and lower extremities to the central circulation.

(b) PASG prevents all blood from flowing to the legs and diminishes blood flow to the pelvis and abdomen, thereby increasing the amount of blood available to the central circulation.

(c) PASG may increase peripheral vascular resistance, which prevents dilation of blood vessels in the lower extremities, thereby protecting the volume of the central circulation.

(d) PASG provides direct pressure to tamponade bleeding in the lower extremities and may diminish blood loss into the abdomen and pelvis.

(e) PASG stabilizes fractures of the pelvis and lower extremities.

119. Inflation of anti-shock trousers can cause all of the following, except

(a) pulmonary edema.

(b) nausea and vomiting.

(c) a decreased amount of bleeding in areas not covered by the garment.

(d) dyspnea from decreased room for chest and diaphragm expansion.

(e) increased injury or tissue damage in cases of lower rib or diaphragmatic injuries.

120. You should apply military anti-shock trousers (MAST) if the trauma patient exhibits any of the following, except

(a) a blood pressure of less than 80 systolic with no other clinical signs or symptoms of shock.

(b) signs and symptoms of abdominal injury.

(c) a blood pressure of 98 systolic, tachycardia, and cool, pale, diaphoretic skin.

(d) signs and symptoms of severe, isolated head injury.

(e) signs and symptoms of pelvic or femoral fractures.

121. Which of the following statements regarding MAST application is false?

(a) MAST may be used on the pregnant trauma patient, but only the legs should be inflated.

(b) In cases of severe shock, the physician may order all 3 compartments of MAST inflated for the pregnant trauma patient.

    (c) Use of MAST may improve the effectiveness of CPR.

    (d) Use of MAST may improve CHF patients who are hypertensive.

    (e) Use of MAST may be indicated in hypotensive anaphylactic shock patients.

122. In cases of profound shock, the EMT should consider requesting a physician's order to

    (a) inflate MAST in the presence of pulmonary edema.

    (b) remove an impaled object from the abdomen, pelvis, or legs and to inflate all 3 compartments of MAST.

    (c) inflate all 3 compartments of MAST on an eviscerated patient.

    (d) All of the above.

    (e) None of the above.

123. Inflation of MAST/PASG is discontinued when

    (a) the patient's blood pressure stabilizes at 100 to 110 systolic.

    (b) the velcro slips.

    (c) the pop-off valves release.

    (d) any of the above occurs.

    (e) None of the above.

124. Which of the following statements regarding functions of the skin is false?

    (a) Skin functions to protect the body from penetration of bacteria and germs.

    (b) Skin assists the regulation of body temperature: water evaporates from the skin surface in cold weather, and the skin's blood vessels constrict in hot weather.

    (c) Skin prevents loss of body fluids and protects underlying structures from minor trauma.

    (d) All of the above are false.

    (e) None of the above is false.

125. The _____ contains sweat glands, sebaceous glands, and hair follicles.

    (a) subcutaneous tissue

    (b) dermis

    (c) epidermis

    (d) All of the above.

    (e) None of the above.

126. The _____ is the outermost layer of skin, consisting of dead cells constantly being rubbed off and replaced.

    (a) subcutaneous tissue
    (b) dermis
    (c) epidermis
    (d) All of the above.
    (e) None of the above.

127. The skin layer composed largely of fat is the _____.

    (a) subcutaneous tissue
    (b) dermis
    (c) epidermis
    (d) All of the above.
    (e) None of the above.

128. A deeper part of the _____ contains cells with some pigment granules to provide skin color characteristics.

    (a) subcutaneous tissue
    (b) dermis
    (c) epidermis
    (d) All of the above.
    (e) None of the above.

129. The _____ serves as the body's layer of insulation.

    (a) subcutaneous tissue
    (b) dermis
    (c) epidermis
    (d) All of the above.
    (e) None of the above.

130. Blood vessels and specialized nerve endings are located in the _____.

    (a) subcutaneous tissue
    (b) dermis
    (c) epidermis
    (d) All of the above.
    (e) None of the above.

131. An injury in which the skin is not broken, but is only bruised, is called

    (a) erythema.
    (b) ecchymosis.
    (c) an abrasion.
    (d) jaundice.
    (e) a contusion.

132. The color of a bruise is called
   (a) erythema.
   (b) ecchymosis.
   (c) an abrasion.
   (d) jaundice.
   (e) a contusion.

133. The "road rash" that occurs when a body slides over gravel or pavement is a very painful form of
   (a) erythema.
   (b) ecchymosis.
   (c) abrasion.
   (d) jaundice.
   (e) contusion.

134. When a stabbing injury causes both entrance and exit wounds, it is called
   (a) an amputation.
   (b) an avulsion.
   (c) a penetrating puncture wound.
   (d) an abrasion.
   (e) a perforating puncture wound.

135. When a missile enters the body but does not leave it, the injury is called
   (a) an amputation.
   (b) an avulsion.
   (c) a penetrating puncture wound.
   (d) an abrasion.
   (e) a perforating puncture wound.

136. When a crushing or shearing force results in the partial or complete removal of a section of tissue, the injury is called
   (a) an amputation.
   (b) an avulsion.
   (c) a penetrating puncture wound.
   (d) an abrasion.
   (e) a perforating puncture wound.

137. When all or a portion of an extremity is partially or completely severed from the body, it is called

(a) an amputation.

(b) an avulsion.

(c) a penetrating puncture wound.

(d) an abrasion.

(e) a perforating puncture wound.

138. A blunt force may cause

(a) fractured bones and ruptured internal organs.

(b) fractured bone ends and lacerated internal organs.

(c) an open or closed wound.

(d) Answers (b) and (c) only.

(e) Answers (a), (b), and (c).

139. A crushing force may cause

(a) fractured bones and ruptured internal organs.

(b) fractured bone ends and lacerated internal organs.

(c) an open or closed wound.

(d) Answers (b) and (c) only.

(e) Answers (a), (b), and (c).

140. Which of the following statements regarding bandages and dressings is false?

(a) Dressings and bandages function to stop bleeding and to prevent further contamination and infection.

(b) Dressings and bandages will protect the wound from further damage.

(c) A dressing holds a bandage in place better than tape, and should be tight enough to control bleeding without interference with the circulation beyond the wound.

(d) All of the above are false.

(e) None of the above is false.

141. Occlusive dressings should be used for all of the following wounds, except

(a) any open wound of the neck.

(b) any open wound of the groin.

(c) any open wound of the abdomen.

(d) any open wound of the posterior thorax.

(e) any open wound between the neck and the shoulder.

142. Standard treatment for an impaled object includes all of the following, except
    (a) removing a perforating object from the cheek.
    (b) shortening an impaled object to allow transportation of the patient.
    (c) stabilization of the object with bulky dressings.
    (d) removal of the object to apply MAST or PASG.
    (e) use of occlusive dressing prior to bulky dressing on areas of the body requiring occlusive dressings.

143. Care for a partial avulsion or amputation includes all of the following, except
    (a) removal of debris that is not significantly embedded.
    (b) cleansing of exposed tissue with peroxide prior to rinsing with sterile water or saline.
    (c) returning the flap or body part to its normal position of function.
    (d) dressing and bandaging the wound.
    (e) splinting the partially amputated extremity.

144. In the event of the complete removal of tissue or a body part from the patient's body, the EMT should
    (a) prevent the patient from observing the lost part, leave it where it lies, and transport the patient to the hospital before psychogenic shock occurs.
    (b) remove only superficial debris from the part; pack ice around it, place it in a plastic bag, and transport it to the hospital with the patient.
    (c) immerse the part in cold liquid (water or milk) and transport it to the hospital with the patient.
    (d) All of the above.
    (e) None of the above.

145. Exposure or protrusion of abdominal contents from an open wound is called
    (a) evisceration.
    (b) invisceration.
    (c) abdominal profusion.
    (d) parietal protrusion.
    (e) visceral protrusion.

146. Treatment of a patient with exposed or protruding abdominal organs includes all of the following, except

   (a) perform a primary survey prior to treatment of the abdominal wound.
   (b) administer high-flow oxygen by nonrebreather mask.
   (c) if the wound is a flap avulsion, gently gather the viscera back into the abdomen and replace the flap before dressing.
   (d) place an occlusive dressing over the exposed viscera to prevent loss of moisture and heat.
   (e) place a thick dressing or towel over the occlusive dressing to prevent heat loss.

147. The muscle of the heart is considered to be

   (a) voluntary muscle.
   (b) involuntary muscle.
   (c) cardiac muscle.
   (d) Both answers (a) and (b).
   (e) Both answers (b) and (c).

148. The muscles of all hollow internal organs (except the heart) consist of

   (a) voluntary muscle.
   (b) involuntary muscle.
   (c) cardiac muscle.
   (d) Both answers (a) and (b).
   (e) Both answers (b and (c).

149. Smooth muscle is considered to be

   (a) voluntary muscle.
   (b) involuntary muscle.
   (c) cardiac muscle.
   (d) Both answers (a) and (b).
   (e) Both answers (b) and (c).

150. Skeletal muscle is considered to be

   (a) voluntary muscle.
   (b) involuntary muscle.
   (c) cardiac muscle.
   (d) Both answers (a) and (b).
   (e) Both answers (b) and (c).

151. The diaphragm is considered to be composed of
- (a) voluntary muscle.
- (b) involuntary muscle.
- (c) cardiac muscle.
- (d) Both answers (a) and (b).
- (e) Both answers (b) and (c).

152. Which of the following is not a function of the skeleton?
- (a) The skeleton gives form to the body.
- (b) The skeleton provides support, permitting us to stand erect.
- (c) Muscles attached to the skeleton provide strength and permit motion at fused joints.
- (d) The skeleton protects the brain and spinal cord.
- (e) The skeleton protects the heart and lungs.

153. The classification of bones includes all of the following, except
- (a) wide bones.
- (b) short bones.
- (c) long bones.
- (d) flat bones.
- (e) irregular bones.

154. The human skeleton normally has _____ bones.
- (a) 106
- (b) 156
- (c) 206
- (d) 215
- (e) 226

155. The axial skeleton consists of all of the following, except
- (a) the skull.
- (b) the ribs.
- (c) the pelvis.
- (d) the sternum.
- (e) the spinal column.

156. The appendicular skeleton consists of all of the following, except
- (a) the clavicles and scapulae.
- (b) the arms, forearms, wrists, hands, and fingers.
- (c) the legs, ankles, feet, and toes.
- (d) the sacrum and coccyx.
- (e) the pelvic bones.

157. The thoracic cavity is enclosed by
   (a) 7 pairs of ribs, 7 thoracic vertebrae, and the sternum.
   (b) 10 pairs of ribs, 10 thoracic vertebrae, and the sternum.
   (c) 12 pairs of ribs, 12 thoracic vertebrae, and the sternum.
   (d) 13 pairs of ribs, 13 thoracic vertebrae, and the sternum.
   (e) 14 pairs of ribs, 14 thoracic vertebrae, and the sternum.

158. In laymen's terms, the _____ is called the shoulder blade.
   (a) ulna
   (b) clavicle
   (c) humerus
   (d) radius
   (e) scapula

159. The bone located on the thumb side of the forearm is the
   _____.
   (a) ulna
   (b) clavicle
   (c) humerus
   (d) radius
   (e) scapula

160. The _____ is the bone of the upper arm.
   (a) ulna
   (b) clavicle
   (c) humerus
   (d) radius
   (e) scapula

161. In laymen's terms, the _____ is called the collar bone.
   (a) ulna
   (b) clavicle
   (c) humerus
   (d) radius
   (e) scapula

162. The bone located on the little finger side of the forearm is
   the _____.
   (a) ulna
   (b) clavicle
   (c) humerus
   (d) radius
   (e) scapula

163. In laymen's terms, the _____ is called the kneecap.
    (a) patella
    (b) tibia
    (c) femur
    (d) fibula
    (e) sacrum

164. The pelvis is a bony ring formed by the _____ and two pelvic bones.
    (a) patella
    (b) tibia
    (c) femur
    (d) fibula
    (e) sacrum

165. The _____ is attached to the pelvis at the hip joint.
    (a) patella
    (b) tibia
    (c) femur
    (d) fibula
    (e) sacrum

166. The longest, heaviest, and strongest bone of the body is the _____.
    (a) patella
    (b) tibia
    (c) femur
    (d) fibula
    (e) sacrum

167. The _____ is the bone in the anterior lower leg.
    (a) patella
    (b) tibia
    (c) femur
    (d) fibula
    (e) sacrum

168. The _____ is the bone in the posterior lower leg.
    (a) patella
    (b) tibia
    (c) femur
    (d) fibula
    (e) sacrum

169. The _____ are the bones of the wrist.
- (a) tarsals
- (b) metatarsals
- (c) carpals
- (d) metacarpals
- (e) phalanges

170. The _____ are the bones of the hand.
- (a) tarsals
- (b) metatarsals
- (c) carpals
- (d) metacarpals
- (e) phalanges

171. The _____ are the bones of the fingers.
- (a) tarsals
- (b) metatarsals
- (c) carpals
- (d) metacarpals
- (e) phalanges

172. The _____ are the bones of the ankle.
- (a) tarsals
- (b) metatarsals
- (c) carpals
- (d) metacarpals
- (e) phalanges

173. The _____ are the bones of the foot.
- (a) tarsals
- (b) metatarsals
- (c) carpals
- (d) metacarpals
- (e) phalanges

174. The _____ are the bones of the toes.
- (a) tarsals
- (b) metatarsals
- (c) carpals
- (d) metacarpals
- (e) phalanges

175. A _____ means a break in the bone.
- (a) fracture
- (b) direct force injury
- (c) dislocation
- (d) sprain
- (e) twisting force injury

176. A _____ is the displacement of the bone ends of a joint.
- (a) fracture
- (b) direct force injury
- (c) dislocation
- (d) sprain
- (e) twisting force injury

177. A _____ is a partial tear or stretching injury of a ligament.
- (a) fracture
- (b) direct force injury
- (c) dislocation
- (d) sprain
- (e) twisting force injury

178. When a bone is cracked, but not severed, it is called
- (a) a transverse fracture.
- (b) a comminuted fracture.
- (c) a greenstick fracture.
- (d) an impacted fracture.
- (e) an oblique fracture.

179. When a break travels straight across the bone, it is called
- (a) a transverse fracture.
- (b) a comminuted fracture.
- (c) a greenstick fracture.
- (d) an impacted fracture.
- (e) an oblique fracture.

180. A break that travels across the bone at an angle is called
- (a) a transverse fracture.
- (b) a comminuted fracture.
- (c) a greenstick fracture.
- (d) an impacted fracture.
- (e) an oblique fracture.

181. When an injury causes the bone ends of the broken bone to jam together, it is called
    (a) a transverse fracture.
    (b) a comminuted fracture.
    (c) a greenstick fracture.
    (d) an impacted fracture.
    (e) an oblique fracture.

182. When sections of bone are crushed and fragmented, it is called
    (a) a transverse fracture.
    (b) a comminuted fracture.
    (c) a greenstick fracture.
    (d) an impacted fracture.
    (e) an oblique fracture.

183. Swelling, discoloration, and pain in the shoulder indicate the presence of a
    (a) fracture.
    (b) dislocation.
    (c) sprain.
    (d) Either answer (a) or (b).
    (e) Any of the above.

184. Swelling, deformity, and pain in the ankle indicate the presence of a
    (a) fracture.
    (b) dislocation.
    (c) sprain.
    (d) Either answer (a) or (b).
    (e) Either answer (b) or (c).

185. Any swelling or pain in a joint with an open wound should be treated as if it is a
    (a) fracture.
    (b) dislocation.
    (c) sprain.
    (d) Either answer (a) or (b).
    (e) Either answer (b) or (c).

186. Any swelling or pain in a joint with a closed wound should be treated as if it is a
    (a) fracture.
    (b) dislocation.

(c) sprain.

(d) Either answer (a) or (b).

(e) Either answer (b) or (c).

187. In the presence of a fracture, there may be a grating sound or sensation when movement causes the bone ends to run together. This sound is called

(a) friction rub.

(b) a compound fracture.

(c) crepitus.

(d) crackling.

(e) subcutaneous emphysema.

188. Complications of an extremity fracture include all of the following, except

(a) pinched or severed nerves.

(b) soft tissue damage.

(c) pinched or lacerated blood vessels.

(d) contaminated wounds.

(e) hemiparesis.

189. Which of the following statements regarding splinting is false?

(a) The primary objective for splinting is to prevent motion of bone fragments or dislocated joints.

(b) Splinting may minimize damage to muscles, nerves, or blood vessels caused by broken bone ends.

(c) Splinting may prevent a closed fracture from becoming an open fracture.

(d) Splinting may minimize restriction of blood flow as a result of bone ends pressing against blood vessels.

(e) Splinting may cause an increase in pain by limiting muscle spasm.

190. The general rules for the splinting of any fracture include all of the following, except

(a) expose the injury and check for a distal pulse.

(b) remove all jewelry from the injured limb and secure it on the patient's person.

(c) gently move the deformed section to check for the presence of crepitus.

(d) dress the wound and pad all rigid splints before splinting.

(e) always leave fingers and toes exposed (unless they are injured and require dressing).

191. Care of an angulated fracture includes all of the following, except

(a) expose the site and check for a distal pulse.

(b) gently move the deformed section to check for the presence of crepitus.

(c) gently attempt to straighten the angulation before splinting.

(d) splint the extremity.

(e) recheck the distal pulse after splinting.

192. Which of the following statements regarding fracture splinting is false?

(a) Use gentle traction to straighten an angulated fracture before splinting.

(b) Straighten deformities near a joint with gentle, steady traction unless significant pain or resistance to correction is encountered.

(c) Immobilize the fracture from the joint above to the joint below.

(d) Gently traction a fractured long bone until protruding bones are drawn back into place.

(e) Pad all rigid splints to prevent pressure and discomfort.

193. Which of the following statements regarding upper extremity injury is true?

(a) A "dropped shoulder" may indicate a fractured scapula.

(b) A patient with a dislocated shoulder that "pops back into place" should be encouraged to move and exercise the shoulder to prevent recurrence of the dislocation.

(c) Removing jewelry and watches may place the EMT at risk for allegations of theft; therefore, allow the emergency room staff to perform this task.

(d) All of the above are true.

(e) None of the above is true.

194. Which of the following statements regarding upper extremity immobilization is false?

(a) A sling and swathe are required on all upper extremity injuries.

(b) Place a roll of bandage in the hand of the injured extremity, unless finger fracture prevents position of function.

(c) Use of airsplints requires monitoring to assess for leaks.

(d) Rigid splints may be used in conjunction with a sling and swathe.

(e) An injured finger may be splinted with a tongue depressor or taped to the adjacent finger.

195. Each of the large winglike bones of the pelvis are called

(a) an ischium.

(b) an ilium.

(c) an iliac crest.

(d) a sacrum.

(e) a pubic bone.

196. The most superior aspect of either side of the pelvis is the

(a) ischium.

(b) ilium.

(c) iliac crest.

(d) sacrum.

(e) pubic bone.

197. The inferior portion of either side of the pelvis is the

(a) ischium.

(b) ilium.

(c) iliac crest.

(d) sacrum.

(e) pubic bone.

198. The posterior segment of the pelvis is the

(a) ischium.

(b) ilium.

(c) iliac crest.

(d) sacrum.

(e) pubic bone.

199. The anterior portion of the pelvis is formed by the

(a) ischium.

(b) ilium.

(c) iliac crest.

(d) sacrum.

(e) pubic bones.

200. The pulse that can be found on the medial side of the ankle, just behind the "ankle bone," is the
- (a) popliteal pulse.
- (b) dorsalis pedis pulse.
- (c) posterior fibial pulse.
- (d) medial tibial pulse.
- (e) posterior tibial pulse.

201. The pulse that is found on the top of the foot is the
- (a) popliteal pulse.
- (b) dorsalis pedis pulse.
- (c) posterior fibial pulse.
- (d) medial tibial pulse.
- (e) posterior tibial pulse.

202. The pulse that sometimes is called "the pedal pulse" is the
- (a) popliteal pulse.
- (b) dorsalis pedis pulse.
- (c) posterior fibial pulse.
- (d) medial tibial pulse.
- (e) posterior tibial pulse.

203. Pelvic fractures
- (a) can result in life-threatening blood loss from a severed artery.
- (b) can result in injuries to internal organs.
- (c) will benefit from traction splinting.
- (d) Both answers (a) and (b).
- (e) Both answers (a) and (c).

204. Closed femur fractures
- (a) can result in life-threatening blood loss from a severed artery.
- (b) can result in injuries to internal organs.
- (c) will benefit from traction splinting.
- (d) Both answers (a) and (b).
- (e) Both answers (a) and (c).

205. Open femur fractures
- (a) can result in life-threatening blood loss from a severed artery.
- (b) can result in injuries to internal organs.
- (c) will benefit from traction splinting.
- (d) Both answers (a) and (b).
- (e) Both answers (a) and (c).

206. Emergency care of a patient with suspected pelvic fracture includes all of the following except

    (a) suspect spinal injury and carefully logroll the patient onto a long backboard.

    (b) securely splint the lower extremities to prevent additional pelvic injury or pain.

    (c) anticipate life-threatening shock.

    (d) administer high-flow oxygen by nonrebreather mask.

    (e) if shock is already present, consider use of MAST or PASG for simultaneous immobilization and treatment of shock.

207. _____ may cause the leg to appear shortened.

    (a) An anterior hip dislocation

    (b) A posterior hip dislocation

    (c) A hip fracture

    (d) Either answer (a) or (c).

    (e) Any of the above.

208. _____ usually causes the thigh to stretch out from the side of the body, to lie flat, and to externally rotate away from the body.

    (a) An anterior hip dislocation

    (b) A posterior hip dislocation

    (c) A hip fracture

    (d) Either answer (a) or (c).

    (e) Any of the above.

209. _____ usually causes the thigh to rotate inward toward the body with the knee typically flexed.

    (a) An anterior hip dislocation

    (b) A posterior hip dislocation

    (c) A hip fracture

    (d) Either answer (a) or (c).

    (e) Any of the above.

210. _____ is the most common hip dislocation.

    (a) An anterior hip dislocation

    (b) A posterior hip dislocation

    (c) A hip fracture

    (d) Either answer (a) or (c).

    (e) Any of the above.

211. _____ may cause damage to the sciatic nerve, and the patient may be unable to raise his toes or foot.

(a) An anterior hip dislocation

(b) A posterior hip dislocation

(c) A hip fracture

(d) Either answer (a) or (c).

(e) Any of the above.

212. _____ sometimes causes no visible or palpable deformity.

(a) An anterior hip dislocation

(b) A posterior hip dislocation

(c) A hip fracture

(d) Either answer (a) or (c).

(e) Any of the above.

213. Which of the following statements regarding emergency care for hip fracture or dislocation is false?

(a) If the dislocation spontaneously relocates during treatment, encourage the patient to rotate and flex the joint to prevent muscle spasm and reduce pain.

(b) Use pillows or blankets to pad and support the hips and/or extremities in the position they are found, before splinting.

(c) Always check for distal pulses before and after splinting.

(d) Anticipate signs and symptoms of shock.

(e) Administer high-flow oxygen by nonrebreather mask.

214. Which of the following statements regarding femur fractures is true?

(a) There will always be marked deformity in the area of a femur fracture.

(b) Shock will rarely develop with a closed femur fracture.

(c) The leg should be gently straightened and immobilized with a traction splint.

(d) All of the above are true.

(e) None of the above is true.

215. Which of the following statements regarding fractures and dislocations of the knee is false?

(a) There is usually acute pain and swelling present, frequently with grotesque deformity.

(b) The EMT should never force a deformity straight and should never straighten a deformity if it causes increased pain to do so.

(c) A traction splint may be used to splint injuries to the knee, but never with application of the traction.

(d) All of the above are false.

(e) None of the above is false.

216. As moisture on the skin dries, heat is lost by

(a) conduction.

(b) convection.

(c) evaporation.

(d) respiration.

(e) radiation.

217. At normal room temperature, without the presence of air currents, heat can be lost through exposed skin by

(a) conduction.

(b) convection.

(c) evaporation.

(d) respiration.

(e) radiation.

218. Cold air passing over the body causes heat loss by

(a) conduction.

(b) convection.

(c) evaporation.

(d) respiration.

(e) radiation.

219. In a cold environment, without the presence of air currents, heat can be lost through exposed skin by

(a) conduction.

(b) convection.

(c) evaporation.

(d) respiration.

(e) radiation.

220. Heat and moisture from the lungs are lost during

(a) conduction.

(b) convection.

(c) evaporation.

(d) respiration.

(e) radiation.

221. The most common illness caused by heat

  (a) is heat cramps.
  (b) is heat exhaustion.
  (c) is heat stroke.
  (d) Both answers (a) and (b).
  (e) Both answers (b) and (c).

222. Strenuous exercise, even in a temperate environment, may produce

  (a) heat cramps.
  (b) heat exhaustion.
  (c) heat stroke.
  (d) Either answer (a) or (b).
  (e) Any of the above.

223. _____ occur(s) when the patient works hard in a hot environment.

  (a) Heat cramps
  (b) Heat exhaustion
  (c) Heat stroke
  (d) Both answers (a) and (b).
  (e) Both answers (b) and (c).

224. _____ cause(s) brain cell injury, and the patient may die.

  (a) Heat cramps
  (b) Heat exhaustion
  (c) Heat stroke
  (d) Both answers (a) and (b).
  (e) Both answers (b) and (c).

225. Painful muscle spasms in the extremities accompany

  (a) heat cramps.
  (b) heat exhaustion.
  (c) heat stroke.
  (d) Both answers (a) and (b).
  (e) Answers (a), (b), and (c).

226. Complaints of weakness accompany

  (a) heat cramps.
  (b) heat exhaustion.
  (c) heat stroke.
  (d) Both answers (b) and (c).
  (e) Answers (a), (b), and (c).

227. The patient with _____ has warm, moist, pink skin.
   (a) heat cramps
   (b) heat exhaustion
   (c) heat stroke
   (d) Both answers (a) and (b).
   (e) None of the above.

228. The patient with _____ has cool, dry, pale skin.
   (a) heat cramps
   (b) heat exhaustion
   (c) heat stroke
   (d) Both answers (a) and (b).
   (e) None of the above.

229. The patient with _____ has cool, moist, pale skin.
   (a) heat cramps
   (b) heat exhaustion
   (c) heat stroke
   (d) Both answers (a) and (b).
   (e) None of the above.

230. The patient with _____ has hot, dry, red skin.
   (a) heat cramps
   (b) heat exhaustion
   (c) heat stroke
   (d) Both answers (b) and (c).
   (e) None of the above.

231. Diaphoresis is present when the patient is suffering from
   (a) heat cramps.
   (b) heat exhaustion.
   (c) heat stroke.
   (d) Both answers (a) and (b).
   (e) Answers (a), (b), and (c).

232. Altered level of consciousness accompanies
   (a) heat cramps.
   (b) heat exhaustion.
   (c) heat stroke.
   (d) Both answers (a) and (b).
   (e) Both answers (b) and (c).

233. Loss of consciousness frequently accompanies
   (a) heat cramps.
   (b) heat exhaustion.
   (c) heat stroke.
   (d) Both answers (a) and (b).
   (e) Both answers (b) and (c).

234. Treatment for heat cramps includes
   (a) giving the conscious patient an electrolyte beverage to drink.
   (b) providing supplemental oxygen and gradual cooling (without causing the patient to shiver).
   (c) providing supplemental oxygen and rapid cooling with wrapped ice packs placed at each side of the neck, in each armpit, at each wrist and ankle, at the groin, and behind each knee.
   (d) Both answers (a) and (b).
   (e) Both answers (a) and (c).

235. Treatment for heat exhaustion includes
   (a) giving the conscious patient an electrolyte beverage to drink.
   (b) providing supplemental oxygen and gradual cooling (without causing the patient to shiver).
   (c) providing supplemental oxygen and rapid cooling with wrapped ice packs placed at each side of the neck, in each armpit, at each wrist and ankle, at the groin, and behind each knee.
   (d) Both answers (a) and (b).
   (e) Both answers (a) and (c).

236. Treatment for heat stroke includes
   (a) giving the conscious patient an electrolyte beverage to drink.
   (b) providing supplemental oxygen and gradual cooling (without causing the patient to shiver).
   (c) providing supplemental oxygen and rapid cooling with wrapped ice packs placed at each side of the neck, in each armpit, at each wrist and ankle, at the groin, and behind each knee.
   (d) Both answers (a) and (b).
   (e) Both answers (a) and (c).

237. The risk of hypothermia is greatly increased in all of the following situations, except

    (a) when the patient's clothing becomes wet.

    (b) when the cold environment is also windy.

    (c) when the patient is elderly or injured.

    (d) when the patient tries to "walk off the chill."

    (e) when the patient drinks alcohol to warm himself.

238. Which of the following statements regarding local cooling of body parts is false?

    (a) When the body is subjected to excessive cold, the water in the cells will freeze.

    (b) Ice crystals that form in the frozen body cells may destroy them.

    (c) If the freezing body part is gently rubbed, the friction heat will melt the ice crystals and greatly diminish the damage caused by freezing.

    (d) All of the above are false.

    (e) None of the above is false.

239. If the patient's skin is cold, white, or gray and feels hard throughout, _____ has occurred.

    (a) frostnip

    (b) superficial frostnip

    (c) deep frostnip

    (d) superficial frostbite

    (e) deep frostbite

240. If the patient's skin is cold, soft, and pliant but blanched, _____ has occurred.

    (a) frostnip

    (b) superficial frostnip

    (c) deep frostnip

    (d) superficial frostbite

    (e) deep frostbite

241. If the patient's skin is cold, white, and waxy, firm to the touch but with soft tissue beneath the surface, _____ has occurred.

    (a) frostnip

    (b) superficial frostnip

    (c) deep frostnip

    (d) superficial frostbite

    (e) deep frostbite

242. Treatment for frostnip includes

    (a) warming the skin with hot breath or firm pressure with a warm hand.

    (b) wrapping the part with dry, sterile dressing and covering the part with blankets.

    (c) resting the part on the bottom of a tub of hot water, adding more hot water as needed.

    (d) Any of the above.

    (e) None of the above.

243. Treatment for frostbite includes

    (a) warming the skin with hot breath or firm pressure with a warm hand.

    (b) wrapping the part with dry, sterile dressing and covering the part with blankets.

    (c) resting the part on the bottom of a tub of hot water, adding more hot water as needed.

    (d) Any of the above.

    (e) None of the above.

244. Which of the following statements regarding treatment of frostbite is true?

    (a) Although cigarette smoking is never encouraged, if transport is delayed allow the patient to smoke if it will calm him down.

    (b) EMTs are not allowed to administer pain medications, but if transport is delayed allow the patient to drink moderate amounts of alcohol to alleviate some of the intense pain that occurs during warming.

    (c) Do not warm or thaw a frozen part if there is any possibility that it will be subjected to cold temperatures again; leave it frozen.

    (d) If the feet have been frozen but are now thawed, assist the patient to walk about to encourage circulation.

    (e) Allow the patient to take his own prescription pain medication before beginning the warming process.

245. Shivering is

    (a) a form of fine muscle tremors that produces chilling of the body.

    (b) a minor form of petit mal seizure caused by the brain's reaction to fear.

    (c) a late sign of hypothermia.

    (d) an attempt by the body to generate heat.

    (e) caused by the irritation of hair follicles, which are sensitive to cold.

246. The earliest signs and symptoms of hypothermia include all of the following, except

    (a) shivering.

    (b) feelings of numbness.

    (c) decreased muscle function.

    (d) drowsiness, unwillingness to do simple tasks.

    (e) slow pulse and slow respiration rate.

247. Various stages of hypothermia produce all of the following signs and symptoms, except

    (a) intense hunger.

    (b) decreased level of conscious.

    (c) failing eyesight.

    (d) freezing body parts.

    (e) apparent death.

248. Which of the following statements regarding severe hypothermia patients is false?

    (a) Ventricular fibrillation may occur even when a patient is rewarmed slowly.

    (b) Ventricular fibrillation may occur with rough handling.

    (c) CPR should be delayed until the patient is warm, to prevent ventricular fibrillation.

    (d) All of the above are false.

    (e) None of the above is false.

249. If less than 30 minutes away from a medical facility, care for the hypothermic patient includes all of the following, except

    (a) prevent further heat loss.

    (b) handle with care and transport rapidly (but gently).

    (c) administer heated oxygen by nonrebreather mask.

    (d) rewarm the patient slowly, placing wrapped heat packs on either side of the neck, at each armpit, at each wrist and ankle, at the groin, and behind each knee.

    (e) perform CPR if the patient suffers cardiopulmonary arrest, regardless of the patient's body temperature.

250. Which of the following statements regarding near-drowning accidents is true?

    (a) Saltwater near-drowning and freshwater near-drowning have different mechanisms of damage to the body.

    (b) Saltwater near-drowning requires suction before pulmonary resuscitation is attempted.

    (c) Freshwater near-drowning requires stronger and deeper ventilations than saltwater near-drowning, to reinflate collapsed alveoli.

    (d) All of the above are true.

    (e) None of the above is true.

251. Which of the following statements regarding near-drowning accidents is false?

    (a) Large amounts of water are swallowed and inhaled during near-drowning; suction the patient before attempting pulmonary resuscitation.

    (b) Direct swimming rescue should be attempted only by personnel trained in water rescue.

    (c) Pulmonary resuscitation should begin immediately, even while the patient is still in the water, but do not begin chest compressions until the patient is out of the water.

    (d) All drowning or near-drowning victims should be treated for potential spine injury.

    (e) All apneic, pulseless patients submerged in cold water should receive resuscitation.

252. All of the following statements regarding near-drowning accidents are true, except

    (a) heart attack or cardiac arrest must be considered as the possible cause of the elderly near-drowning victim.

    (b) near-drowning victims may have a better potential for resuscitation and survival if the water involved was cold.

    (c) the mammalian diving reflex provides some protection for the heart and brain in warm-water near-drowning accidents.

    (d) alcohol and drug abuse may be a factor in near-drownings.

    (e) internal injuries may have occurred before, during, or after the actual near-drowning accident.

253. Which of the following statements regarding air embolism is true?

    (a) Air embolism is generally caused by divers holding their breath, can occur in shallow water, and causes a rapid onset of signs and symptoms.

    (b) When water pressure around the chest is rapidly reduced, the air held within the lungs expands and may rupture alveoli or damage adjacent blood vessels.

    (c) A pneumothorax may develop from alveoli that rupture into the lung cavity; an air embolism will develop if the alveoli rupture into the circulatory system.

    (d) An air embolism can travel to the heart or the brain, causing serious injury or death.

    (e) All of the above are true.

254. Signs and symptoms of air embolism include all of the following, except

    (a) dyspnea with chest pain; froth from the nose or mouth.

    (b) intense hunger.

    (c) pain in the muscles, joints, tendons, abdomen; blotching or itching of the skin.

    (d) dizziness, vomiting, and/or vision difficulties.

    (e) possible paralysis and unconsciousness.

255. Which of the following statements regarding decompression sickness is true?

    (a) The nitrogen concentration in room air is greater than that of oxygen, and nitrogen is carried in the blood in small bubbles that are slowly released into the tissues.

    (b) In a rapid ascent from a deep dive, the pressure around the chest is released quickly and the nitrogen bubbles become larger, possibly obstructing the vessels or body tissues in which they lie.

    (c) The signs and symptoms of decompression sickness develop slowly, and the patient may not seek help for up to 24 hours after the actual incident.

    (d) All of the above are true.

    (e) None of the above is true.

256. Signs and symptoms of decompression sickness include
  (a) severe pain in the muscles and joints (called "the bends").
  (b) fatigue or altered level of consciousness.
  (c) dyspnea, chest pain, choking, coughing or frothy blood-tinged sputum.
  (d) skin rashes, numbness, or paralysis.
  (e) Any or all of the above, prior to unconsciousness or death.

257. Treatment of patients with air embolism or decompression sickness includes
  (a) basic life support and high-flow oxygen.
  (b) placing the patient in the left laterally recumbent position on a long backboard, and elevation of the foot end of the board.
  (c) transportation of the patient to the medical facility, preferably one with a hyperbaric oxygen (HBO) chamber.
  (d) All of the above.
  (e) None of the above.

The answer key for Test Section Three is on page 224.

4

Test
Section
Four

Test Section Four covers the following subjects and their treatment:

* Injuries to the Head, Face, Eyes, Neck and Spine
* Injuries to the Chest, Abdomen and Genitalia
* Emergency Childbirth
* Burns (Heat, Chemical, Electrical, Radiation)
* Hazardous Materials
* Psychological Aspects of Emergency Care
* Medical Terminology

EMT - Basic
National Standards Review Self Test

1.   The axial skeleton consists of
     (a) the skull and spine.
     (b) the skull, spine, ribs, and sternum.
     (c) the skull, spine, ribs, sternum, and clavicles.
     (d) the skull, spine, ribs, sternum, clavicles, and pelvis.
     (e) the skull, spine, and pelvis.

2.   The rib cage includes
     (a) the ribs.
     (b) the ribs and sternum.
     (c) the ribs, sternum, and thoracic vertebrae.
     (d) the ribs, sternum, thoracic vertebrae, and clavicles.
     (e) the ribs, sternum, thoracic vertebrae, clavicles, and
          scapulae.

3.   The thoracic spine consists of how many vertebrae?
     (a) 4
     (b) 5
     (c) 7
     (d) 10
     (e) 12

4.   The lumbar spine consists of how many vertebrae?
     (a) 4
     (b) 5
     (c) 7
     (d) 10
     (e) 12

5.   The sacrum consists of how many fused vertebrae?
     (a) 4
     (b) 5
     (c) 7
     (d) 10
     (e) 12

6.   The cervical spine consists of how many vertebrae?
     (a) 4
     (b) 5
     (c) 7

      (d) 10

      (e) 12

7. The coccyx consists of how many fused vertebrae?

      (a) 4

      (b) 5

      (c) 7

      (d) 10

      (e) 12

8. A patient with a fractured jaw has a fractured

      (a) zygomatic bone.

      (b) scapula.

      (c) mandible.

      (d) ethmoid.

      (e) sternum.

9. A patient with a fractured breastbone has a fractured

      (a) zygomatic bone.

      (b) scapula.

      (c) mandible.

      (d) ethmoid.

      (e) sternum.

10. A patient with a fractured cheekbone has a fractured

      (a) zygomatic bone.

      (b) scapula.

      (c) mandible.

      (d) ethmoid.

      (e) sternum.

11. The nervous system consists of

      (a) the brain.

      (b) the spinal cord.

      (c) nerves entering and leaving the brain and spinal cord.

      (d) Answers (a) and (b) only.

      (e) All of the above.

12. The central nervous system consists of

      (a) the brain.

      (b) the spinal cord.

      (c) nerves entering and leaving the brain and spinal cord.

      (d) Answers (a) and (b) only.

      (e) All of the above.

13.   The peripheral nervous system consists of
   (a)   the brain.
   (b)   the spinal cord.
   (c)   nerves entering and leaving the brain and spinal cord.
   (d)   Answers (a) and (b) only.
   (e)   All of the above.

14.   Nerves that send information to the brain on what the different parts of the body are doing relative to their surroundings are called
   (a)   cerebral nerves.
   (b)   skeletal nerves.
   (c)   sensory nerves.
   (d)   motor nerves.
   (e)   spinal nerves.

15.   Nerves that emanate from the brain and result in stimulation of a muscle or organ are called
   (a)   cerebral nerves.
   (b)   skeletal nerves.
   (c)   sensory nerves.
   (d)   motor nerves.
   (e)   spinal nerves.

16.   Which of the following statements regarding the autonomic nervous system is false?
   (a)   The autonomic nervous system can slow or increase the heart rate.
   (b)   The autonomic nervous system can constrict or dilate blood vessels.
   (c)   The autonomic nervous system can constrict or dilate the bronchi of the lungs.
   (d)   All of the above are false.
   (e)   None of the above is false.

17.   Which of the following statements regarding the brain is false?
   (a)   The brain is the controlling organ of the body and the center of consciousness.
   (b)   The spinal cord is the only link between the brain and the body.
   (c)   The brain occupies the entire space within the cranium.
   (d)   Each type of brain cell has a specific function.
   (e)   Certain parts of the brain perform certain functions.

18. Which of the following statements regarding skull fractures is false?
     (a) Fractures of the skull are common in accident victims.
     (b) Their seriousness depends on the amount of injury to the brain.
     (c) Serious brain injury is much more common when there is not a skull fracture present.
     (d) All of the above are false.
     (e) None of the above is false.

19. The most common skull fracture is the
     (a) linear skull fracture.
     (b) comminuted skull fracture.
     (c) depressed skull fracture.
     (d) penetrated skull.
     (e) basal skull fracture.

20. A direct blow to the top of the posterior neck can cause a
     (a) linear skull fracture.
     (b) comminuted skull fracture.
     (c) depressed skull fracture.
     (d) penetrated skull.
     (e) basal skull fracture.

21. When an injury causes pieces of the skull to be pushed inward, pressing on or injuring the brain, the patient has a
     (a) linear skull fracture.
     (b) comminuted skull fracture.
     (c) depressed skull fracture.
     (d) penetrated skull.
     (e) basal skull fracture.

22. When an injury produces multiple cracks in the skull that radiate from the point of impact, the patient has a
     (a) linear skull fracture.
     (b) comminuted skull fracture.
     (c) depressed skull fracture.
     (d) penetrated skull.
     (e) basal skull fracture.

23. A thin crack in the skull is called a

  (a) linear skull fracture.
  (b) comminuted skull fracture.
  (c) depressed skull fracture.
  (d) penetrated skull.
  (e) basal skull fracture.

24. When objects such as bullets or knives pass through the skull, causing direct brain injury, the patient is described as having a

  (a) linear skull fracture.
  (b) comminuted skull fracture.
  (c) depressed skull fracture.
  (d) penetrated skull.
  (e) basal skull fracture.

25. A cerebral concussion is defined as

  (a) bleeding and abnormal swelling of brain tissue.
  (b) a temporary loss of function for some or all of the brain.
  (c) blood clots causing pressure on brain tissue.
  (d) All of the above.
  (e) None of the above.

26. A cerebral contusion is defined as

  (a) bleeding and abnormal swelling of brain tissue.
  (b) a temporary loss of function for some or all of the brain.
  (c) blood clots causing pressure on brain tissue.
  (d) All of the above.
  (e) None of the above.

27. A cerebral hematoma is defined as

  (a) bleeding and abnormal swelling of brain tissue.
  (b) a temporary loss of function for some or all of the brain.
  (c) blood clots causing pressure on brain tissue.
  (d) All of the above.
  (e) None of the above.

28. Which of the following statements regarding a cerebral concussion is false?

  (a) The patient may be confused or may have a staggering gait.
  (b) The patient may lose consciousness.

     (c) Paralysis may be present on one side of the body or in all four limbs.

     (d) All of the above are false.

     (e) None of the above is false.

29. Which of the following statements regarding a cerebral contusion is false?

     (a) The patient may be confused or may have a staggering gait.

     (b) The patient may lose consciousness.

     (c) Paralysis may be present on one side of the body or in all four limbs.

     (d) All of the above are false.

     (e) None of the above is false.

30. Loss of memory for the events surrounding an accident or injury is called

     (a) amniosis.

     (b) senility.

     (c) amnesia.

     (d) Alzheimers.

     (e) stupor.

31. Which of the following statements regarding facial fracture is true?

     (a) Facial fractures are always serious and disfiguring injuries and can cause psychological distress.

     (b) Because of their painful nature, facial fractures rarely go undetected.

     (c) Unless there is a secondary impact, skull fractures rarely accompany facial fractures.

     (d) All of the above are true.

     (e) None of the above is true.

32. A subdural hematoma results when head injury causes blood to collect or pool

     (a) between the meninges and the skull.

     (b) between the brain and the meninges.

     (c) within the brain tissue.

     (d) behind the eyes.

     (e) behind the ears or at the base of the skull.

33.   An epidural hematoma results when head injury causes
            blood to collect or pool
            (a) between the meninges and the skull.
            (b) between the brain and the meninges.
            (c) within the brain tissue.
            (d) behind the eyes.
            (e) behind the ears or at the base of the skull.

34.   An intracerebral hematoma results when head injury
            causes blood to collect or pool
            (a) between the meninges and the skull.
            (b) between the brain and the meninges.
            (c) within the brain tissue.
            (d) behind the eyes.
            (e) behind the ears or at the base of the skull.

35.   Battle's sign is defined as bruising
            (a) between the meninges and the skull.
            (b) between the brain and the meninges.
            (c) within the brain tissue.
            (d) behind the eyes.
            (e) behind the ears or at the base of the skull.

36.   Raccoon's sign is defined as bruising
            (a) between the meninges and the skull.
            (b) between the brain and the meninges.
            (c) within the brain tissue.
            (d) behind the eyes.
            (e) behind the ears or at the base of the skull.

37.   Signs of a skull fracture include all but which of the follow-
            ing signs?
            (a) Deformity of the skull.
            (b) Blood or clear fluid draining from the ears or nose.
            (c) The bull's-eye sign.
            (d) Raccoon's eyes.
            (e) Battle's sign.

38.   Which of the following statements regarding raccoon's eyes
            and Battle's sign is true?
            (a) Raccoon's eyes indicate a skull fracture only.
            (b) Battle's sign occurs only when a direct blow strikes the
                skull behind the ears.

(c) Facial fractures are frequently associated with Battle's sign.

(d) Raccoon's eyes and Battle's sign require time to develop and therefore may not be present.

(e) Raccoon's eyes and Battle's sign are not reliable indicators of the presence or lack of skull fracture, and therefore should not be charted.

39. The brain and spinal cord are protected by layers of tissue filled with a clear liquid called

(a) crainiospinal fluid.
(b) cerebrospinal fluid.
(c) crainialdural fluid.
(d) intracerebral fluid.
(e) epiduralcerebral fluid.

40. Which of the following statements regarding this protective fluid is false?

(a) This fluid also serves as a shock absorber to diminish injury to the brain tissue.
(b) This fluid also provides nutrition to some of the brain cells.
(c) When a skull fracture is present, this fluid and blood may drain from the nose or ears.
(d) All of the above are false.
(e) None of the above is false.

41. Which of the following statements regarding care for a skull fracture is true?

(a) Do not attempt to stop bleeding from the nose or ears when a skull fracture is suspected.
(b) It is vital to stop any bleeding from the nose or ears to prevent hypovolemia.
(c) If bleeding from the nose or ears is not stopped, an infection around the brain will occur.
(d) If bleeding from the nose or ears is not stopped, increased pressure on the brain will occur.
(e) Both answers (c) and (d) are true.

42. As an isolated head injury becomes worse, increased intercrainial pressure will cause
    (a) an increase in blood pressure and heart rate.
    (b) an increase in blood pressure and a decreased heart rate.
    (c) a decrease in blood pressure and heart rate.
    (d) a decrease in blood pressure and an increased heart rate.
    (e) little change as the blood pressure is unable to increase or decrease due to brain damage.

43. Elements included in the Glasgow Coma Scale evaluation of a trauma patient's motor response do not include
    (a) seizure activity (1 point).
    (b) extension response to painful stimuli (2 points).
    (c) flexion response to painful stimuli (3 points).
    (d) withdrawal from painful stimuli (4 points).
    (e) localizing painful stimuli (5 points).

44. When reporting the verbal responses of a patient with a head injury, the EMT should specify whether the patient is
    (a) oriented to person, place, and time or is semi-comatose.
    (b) alert and oriented or obtunded and lethargic.
    (c) awake or comatose.
    (d) All of the above.
    (e) None of the above.

45. The EMT should oxygenate the patient with a head injury using
    (a) a nasal cannula at 4 LPM if the patient has a history of COPD.
    (b) a nonrebreather mask at 6 LPM.
    (c) bag-valve-mask assist at 15 LPM and a rate of 25 or more ventilations per minute if the patient becomes unconscious.
    (d) All of the above.
    (e) None of the above.

46. Which of the following statements regarding care for patients with a head injury and suspected c-spine fracture is false?
    (a) Maintain respiration and circulation.
    (b) Use a long backboard or similar immobilization device, despite the patient's denial of spine pain.

(c) Control bleeding, but not from the nose or ears.

(d) Elevate the head of the long backboard if shock is not present.

(e) Apply soft extremity restraints for patient protection in the event of convulsions.

47. The most serious potential complication of facial fractures is

(a) obstruction of the airway.

(b) permanent facial disfiguration.

(c) associated spinal fractures and spinal cord damage.

(d) associated skull fractures and brain damage.

(e) permanent blindness.

48. Which of the following statements regarding objects impaled in the skull is true?

(a) An object impaled in the skull must be removed to prevent further brain damage.

(b) The rigid skull will stabilize any impaled object. Therefore, the object should remain in place and no additional time should be wasted on additional stabilization.

(c) An object impaled in the skull indicates irreversible brain injury and will lead to disability or death despite any actions the EMT may take.

(d) All of the above are true.

(e) None of the above is true.

49. If your patient has a potential spine injury and is wearing a football helmet, which of the following statements is true?

(a) Removal of the helmet is mandatory in any case.

(b) If the airway can be accessed and managed with the helmet on, it may remain on.

(c) Removing a helmet is a simple skill and can be carefully accomplished by one EMT.

(d) The patient must be immobilized on a spine board prior to removal of the helmet.

(e) A cervical collar must be in place prior to removal of the helmet.

50. Which of the following statements regarding spinal injuries is true?

    (a) A lack of sensation or inability to move some or all body parts will always be present.

    (b) The patient will always deny pain at the site of the injury.

    (c) The patient will never have feeling below the site of the injury.

    (d) The mechanism of injury will always indicate the presence of spine injury.

    (e) The mechanism of injury is frequently the only indicator of the presence of spine injury.

51. An EMT should suspect a spinal cord injury in the patient who

    (a) is involved in a diving accident.

    (b) jumped from a second-story window to land on both feet in the grass.

    (c) received a small caliber gunshot wound to the head.

    (d) All of the above.

    (e) None of the above.

52. Which of the following statements regarding complications of neck injuries is false?

    (a) Neck injuries may cause inadequate breathing.

    (b) Neck injuries may cause paralysis of the nerves affecting the size of the blood vessels.

    (c) Shock may result from neck injuries.

    (d) Neck injuries are rarely the subject of lawsuits.

    (e) Neck injuries are only sometimes accompanied by pain.

53. Which of the following statements regarding the management and evaluation of an unconscious trauma patient is false?

    (a) Airway management and support are always the first priority.

    (b) Bleeding control may be accomplished by compressing the scalp against the skull if there is no indication of skull fracture.

    (c) Observe positioning of arms and legs upon approach.

    (d) Start with the hands to evaluate presence of sensation by pinching the anterior of each hand.

    (e) Observe the male patient for presence of priapism.

54. Which of the following statements regarding spinal immobilization is false?

    (a) Always realign the spine with gentle traction before immobilization.

    (b) Immobilization should occur before moving the patient to the ambulance.

    (c) Always fully immobilize the unconscious trauma patient.

    (d) All of the above are false.

    (e) None of the above is false.

55. Injuries to the face and scalp

    (a) rarely bleed heavily unless serious injury has occurred.

    (b) benefit from direct pressure, especially when placed over a fracture site.

    (c) may prove fatal if an artery is severed.

    (d) require removal of debris and protruding pieces to protect the airway.

    (e) should be covered with occlusive dressings.

56. Which of the following statements regarding care of scalp wounds is false?

    (a) An EMT should clean or clear the surface of the wound so that debris will not be imbedded further when the wound is dressed.

    (b) Cover exposed nerves, tendons, or blood vessels with a moist sterile dressing.

    (c) Apply gentle pressure to the wound with a dry sterile dressing to control bleeding.

    (d) All of the above are false.

    (e) None of the above is false.

57. Which of the following statements regarding care for facial trauma is true?

    (a) Cover exposed nerves, tendons, or blood vessels with a moist sterile dressing.

    (b) Flaps of partially avulsed skin should be returned to their normal position before bandaging.

    (c) Skin sections that are fully avulsed should be wrapped in dry sterile dressing, sealed in a plastic bag, and placed on ice for transport.

    (d) All of the above are true.

    (e) None of the above is true.

58. Which of the following statements regarding care for an object that is impaled and perforates the cheek is true?

(a) Gently remove the object and pack roller gauze between the teeth and cheek.

(b) Do not remove the impaled object; stabilize it with occlusive dressing and monitor the airway closely.

(c) Gently remove the object, but do not pack the inside of the cheek. To do so may cause airway obstruction with vomitus or packing material.

(d) Do not remove the impaled object; stabilize it with a bulky dressing and monitor the airway closely.

(e) If gentle traction does not remove the object, make one attempt to gently twist the object free. Then pack roller gauze between the teeth and cheek, leaving 3 to 4 inches of gauze outside of the patient's mouth.

59. The anterior chamber of the eye is filled with a clear liquid called

(a) visceral humor.
(b) aqueous humor.
(c) vitreous humor.
(d) aquial humor.
(e) globular gel.

60. The posterior chamber of the eye is filled with a clear, gellike substance called the

(a) visceral humor.
(b) aqueous humor.
(c) vitreous humor.
(d) aquial humor.
(e) globular gel.

61. Liquid lost from the anterior chamber due to an eye injury

(a) can be replaced by the body.
(b) can be replaced by a prosthetic gel.
(c) can be replaced by a synthetic humor.
(d) can be replaced by a synthetic gel.
(e) cannot be replaced by the body.

62. Gel lost from the posterior chamber due to an eye injury

(a) can be replaced by the body.
(b) can be replaced by a prosthetic gel.
(c) can be replaced by a synthetic humor.
(d) can be replaced by a synthetic gel.
(e) cannot be replaced by the body.

63.   The white area of the eye is called the

    (a) iris.
    (b) cornea.
    (c) sclera.
    (d) conjunctiva.
    (e) lens.

64.   The colored area of the eye is called the

    (a) iris.
    (b) cornea.
    (c) sclera.
    (d) conjunctiva.
    (e) lens.

65.   The membrane that lines the undersurfaces of the eyelids is called the

    (a) iris.
    (b) cornea.
    (c) sclera.
    (d) conjunctiva.
    (e) lens.

66.   The protective clear covering of the anterior eye assists in focusing light and is called the

    (a) iris.
    (b) cornea.
    (c) sclera.
    (d) conjunctiva.
    (e) lens.

67.   The anterior and posterior chambers of the eye are separated by the

    (a) iris.
    (b) cornea.
    (c) sclera.
    (d) conjunctiva.
    (e) lens.

68.   Bright light causes the pupil of the eye to become

    (a) unequal.
    (b) dilated.
    (c) swollen.
    (d) constricted.
    (e) fixed.

69.   Darkness causes the pupil of the eye to become
       (a) unequal.
       (b) dilated.
       (c) swollen.
       (d) constricted.
       (e) fixed.

70.   Emergency care of an injured eye includes
       (a) leaving the uninjured eye uncovered to prevent anxiety
           or hysteria.
       (b) application of direct pressure to prevent loss of ocular
           fluid or gel.
       (c) removal of small bodies lodged on the cornea to prevent
           blindness.
       (d) All of the above.
       (e) None of the above.

71.   Movement of the eyes is directly linked and coordinated.
       When one eye moves, the other moves in precisely the same
       manner. This cannot be altered voluntarily and is called
       (a) sympathetic eye movement.
       (b) involuntary eye movement.
       (c) paradoxical eye movement.
       (d) empathetic eye movement.
       (e) parathetic eye movement.

72.   When chemical burns of the eye are treated,
       (a) both eyes should be flushed with water for 20 to 30
           minutes.
       (b) both eyes should be covered with a dry sterile dressing.
       (c) both eyes should be covered with a moist sterile
           dressing.
       (d) the affected eye should be flushed with water for 20 to
           30 minutes.
       (e) the injured eye should be covered with a moist sterile
           dressing.

73.   When a burned eyelid is treated,
       (a) both eyes should be flushed with water for 20 to 30
           minutes.
       (b) both eyes should be covered with a dry sterile dressing.
       (c) both eyes should be covered with a moist sterile
           dressing.
       (d) the affected eye should be flushed with water for 20 to
           30 minutes.

(e) the injured eye should be covered with a moist sterile dressing.

74. When light burns to the eyes are treated,
(a) both eyes should be flushed with water for 20 to 30 minutes.
(b) both eyes should be covered with a dry sterile dressing.
(c) both eyes should be covered with a moist sterile dressing.
(d) the affected eye should be flushed with water for 20 to 30 minutes.
(e) the injured eye should be covered with a moist sterile dressing.

75. When one is managing a patient with an object impaled in the eye, which of the following statements is true?
(a) The uninjured eye should remain uncovered to reduce eye movement.
(b) Remove the object and apply an occlusive dressing to prevent loss of ocular fluid or gel.
(c) Stabilize the object in place with gauze and a protective paper cup.
(d) Irrigate the object with sterile saline to prevent infection.
(e) Apply an ocular antibiotic prior to stabilization with bulky dressings to prevent infection.

76. When one is caring for an eye-injured patient who is wearing contact lenses, which of the following statements is false?
(a) If a corrosive substance has been splashed in the eye, a contact lens may prevent successful irrigation and promote further injuries.
(b) Contact lenses must be removed in the presence of obvious injury to prevent further eye injury.
(c) Unless a corrosive substance is involved, soft contact lenses may remain on the eye.
(d) Specialized suction cups are available for the removal of hard contact lenses.
(e) If you cannot remove the lens, leave it in and slide it onto the white of the eye.

77. An avulsed eye is one that has been
- (a) lacerated so that a flap is created.
- (b) extruded from its socket.
- (c) collapsed from loss of the ocular fluid or gel.
- (d) Any of the above.
- (e) None of the above.

78. When one is managing a patient with an avulsed eye, which of the following statements is true?
- (a) Leave the uninjured eye uncovered to reduce eye movements.
- (b) Replace the flap and cover with an occlusive dressing to control loss of ocular fluid or gel.
- (c) Stabilize the extruded eye with gauze and a protective paper cup.
- (d) Irrigate the eye thouroughly to prevent infection.
- (e) Apply an ocular antibiotic prior to stabilizing with bulky dressings to prevent infection.

79. The ears and their associated structures are responsible for
- (a) hearing.
- (b) hearing and fine muscle coordination.
- (c) hearing and sense of smell.
- (d) hearing and sense of balance.
- (e) hearing and peripheral vision.

80. Complaints of the sensation of a "clogged ear" may indicate
- (a) the presence of a foreign object in the ear.
- (b) a damaged eardrum.
- (c) fluids collecting in the middle ear.
- (d) All of the above.
- (e) None of the above.

81. Children often place toys, beans, or other objects in their noses. If an object can be seen on casual observation of the nose,
- (a) gently pull the object free, using forceps.
- (b) have the patient close the other nostril and forcefully blow his nose.

    (c) have the patient forcefully blow her nose while both nostrils are open.

    (d) have the patient close the other nostril and gently blow his nose.

    (e) leave the object undisturbed and transport the patient to the ER.

82. A serious nosebleed can be caused by

    (a) hypertension or infection.

    (b) excessive sneezing or nose picking.

    (c) brain injury.

    (d) Answers (a) and (c) only.

    (e) All of the above.

83. When oral trauma has produced an avulsed tooth, find the tooth (or tooth part) and

    (a) transport it to the ER with the patient, in a covered container of cold milk.

    (b) gently brush the tooth free of debris and wrap it in a moist sterile dressing before placing it on ice.

    (c) rinse off the tooth, replace it in the socket, cover it with the corner of a moist sterile 4 x 4, and have the patient bite down on it to control socket bleeding.

    (d) Any of the above.

    (e) None of the above.

84. Trauma that involves the neck is

    (a) always considered to be serious.

    (b) considered to be serious only when a spine injury is suspected.

    (c) considered to be serious only when the airway is compromised.

    (d) considered to be serious only when an artery is severed.

    (e) Answers (b), (c), and (d).

85. Signs and symptoms of blunt trauma to the neck may include

    (a) crackling sensations, indicating air under the skin.

    (b) hoarseness or loss of voice.

    (c) airway obstruction.

    (d) Answers (a) and (b) only.

    (e) All of the above.

86. Which of the following statements regarding care for neck wounds is false?

   (a) Control arterial bleeding by direct pressure with a gloved hand.
   (b) If a large vein is torn, apply pressure above and below the point of bleeding to prevent air from entering.
   (c) Apply a circumferential pressure bandage to control bleeding.
   (d) All of the above are false.
   (e) None of the above is false.

87. To dress and bandage bleeding wounds of the neck, use

   (a) a dry sterile dressing with direct pressure.
   (b) an occlusive dressing with direct pressure.
   (c) a moist sterile dressing with direct pressure.
   (d) a dry sterile dressing and avoid any direct pressure.
   (e) an occlusive dressing and avoid any direct pressure.

88. Which of the following statements regarding the bony structure of the chest is true?

   (a) The chest includes 12 thoracic vertebrae.
   (b) The chest includes 10 pairs of ribs connected with cartilage to other ribs or the sternum.
   (c) The chest includes 2 pairs of ribs connected only to the vertebrae.
   (d) All of the above are true.
   (e) None of the above is true.

89. Trauma involving the chest may also cause injuries to

   (a) the heart, major blood vessels, lungs, and trachea.
   (b) the liver and spleen.
   (c) the gallbladder and stomach.
   (d) All of the above.
   (e) None of the above.

90. Which of the following statements regarding chest compression injuries is false?

   (a) A chest compression injury can result from correct application of CPR.
   (b) Chest compression injuries are always closed injuries.

(c) Compression of the chest can increase intrathoracic pressure.

(d) Chest compression injuries may rupture the lungs or heart, and may fracture the ribs or sternum.

(e) Chest compression injuries can result in death.

91. Signs and symptoms of chest injury may include
(a) dyspnea, hemoptysis, cyanosis, tachycardia, hypotension.
(b) hematemesis, bradycardia, hypertension.
(c) dysuria, hematuria, dysrhythmias.
(d) Both answers (a) and (b).
(e) Both answers (a) and (c).

92. Subcutaneous emphysema is defined as
(a) wheezing on inspiration due to air leakage into soft tissues.
(b) wheezing on expiration due to air leakage into soft tissues.
(c) crackling sensations due to air leakage into soft tissues.
(d) rales on inspiration due to air leakage into soft tissues.
(e) rales on expiration due to air leakage into soft tissues.

93. A sucking chest wound can be caused by all of the following except
(a) a stab wound to the left upper quadrant of the abdomen.
(b) a gunshot wound to the base of the neck.
(c) a closed rib fracture from a blunt blow to the back.
(d) a stab wound to the anterior right shoulder.
(e) a gunshot wound to the left armpit.

94. A pneumothorax is defined as
(a) air in the chest cavity from an open chest wound.
(b) air in the chest cavity from a closed chest wound.
(c) pneumonia causing air to be pushed into the chest cavity.
(d) pneumonia causing air to be sucked into the chest cavity.
(e) air in the chest cavity, entering from an open or closed lung laceration.

95. A pneumothorax can be caused by
- (a) a stab wound to the left upper quadrant of the abdomen.
- (b) a closed rib fracture from a blunt blow to the back.
- (c) congenital lung defects, scar tissue from old injuries, or lung cancer.
- (d) All of the above.
- (e) None of the above.

96. Which of the following is not a sign of a simple pneumothorax?
- (a) diminished or absent breath sounds on the injured side.
- (b) distended neck veins.
- (c) uneven chest wall expansion.
- (d) tracheal shift toward the injured side.
- (e) hypotension.

97. Occlusive dressings are used on all open wounds between the chin and the umbilicus to prevent
- (a) air from entering the chest cavity from the atmosphere.
- (b) air from leaving the chest and deflating the lungs.
- (c) blood from leaving the chest and deflating the lungs.
- (d) All of the above.
- (e) None of the above.

98. A tension pneumothorax can be caused by
- (a) a stab wound to the left upper quadrant of the abdomen.
- (b) a closed rib fracture from a blunt blow to the back.
- (c) congenital lung defects, scar tissue from old injuries, or lung cancer.
- (d) All of the above.
- (e) None of the above.

99. Which of the following is not a sign of a tension pneumothorax?
- (a) diminished or absent breath sounds on the injured side.
- (b) distended neck veins.
- (c) uneven chest wall expansion.
- (d) tracheal shift toward the injured side.
- (e) hypotension.

100. Which of the following statements regarding tension pneumothorax is false?
     (a) Release of a bandage covering an open chest wound may be effective in releasing tension.
     (b) Tension pneumothorax can be caused by an EMT sealing an open chest wound.
     (c) A tension pneumothorax can develop again, even after the tension is once released.
     (d) Tension pneumothorax can result in a collapsed lung or a compressed heart.
     (e) A tension pneumothorax will not develop from a closed chest injury.

101. A 24-year-old woman has a screwdriver impaled in her anterior chest, just left lateral to her sternum. You observe that she is apnic. Your best course of action is to
     (a) wrap vaseline gauze around the point of entry and stabilize the screwdriver in place with bulky dressings.
     (b) begin artificial respirations, check her pulse, and stabilize the screwdriver in place with bulky dressings.
     (c) begin artificial respirations, check her pulse, and remove the screwdriver if chest compressions are required so that further damage is avoided.
     (d) remove the screwdriver and seal the wound with occlusive dressing prior to initiating ventilations so that air will not escape around the screwdriver.
     (e) determine if the screwdriver has punctured the heart and treat for cardiac tamponade.

102. Which of the following statements regarding rib fractures is true?
     (a) Rib fracture is a common finding in the presence of trauma and localized chest pain.
     (b) Simple rib fractures should not be bound, strapped, or taped.
     (c) With multiple rib fractures, the patient may be more comfortable with the arm strapped to the chest with a swathe.
     (d) All of the above are true.
     (e) None of the above is true.

103. Failure of one side of the chest to expand normally with inspiration can be caused by all of the following except

  (a) rib fracture.
  (b) flail chest.
  (c) paradoxical respirations.
  (d) penetrating chest injury.
  (e) blunt chest injury.

104. Flail chest is defined as the condition in which

  (a) each rib on one side of the chest has one fracture.
  (b) paradoxical respirations are observed.
  (c) each of three or more ribs is broken in two or more places.
  (d) each of two or more ribs is broken in a different place.
  (e) one-half of the chest does not move with the other.

105. In the presence of an unstable flail segment, paradoxical movement of the chest is described as the chest wall moving

  (a) outward while the flail segment moves inward during inspiration.
  (b) inward while the flail segment moves outward during inspiration.
  (c) outward while the flail segment moves inward during expiration.
  (d) outward while the sternum moves inward during expiration.
  (e) inward while the sternum moves outward during inspiration.

106. A flail segment is best stabilized with

  (a) a 10-lb sandbag secured to the injured side of the chest.
  (b) bulky dressing taped over the site.
  (c) a small pillow held over the site with direct manual pressure.
  (d) Any of the above.
  (e) None of the above.

107. Which of the following statements regarding a flail chest is false?

  (a) Immobilizing the ribs may improve respirations.
  (b) The separation of the sternum from its attachments with the rib cage is another form of flail chest.

(c) CPR frequently causes a flail chest.

(d) A flail chest may be caused by blunt back injury.

(e) A flail section most often occurs at the weaker connections of the ribs to the spine.

108. Which of the following statements regarding a hemothorax is false?

(a) A hemothorax is caused by penetrating, open chest wounds only.

(b) Blood leaking into the chest cavity causes a hemothorax.

(c) Blood leaking into the lung itself causes a hemothorax.

(d) A hemothorax may result in the collapse of a lung.

(e) A hemothorax can result from a lacerated lung or blood vessel.

109. Traumatic asphyxia

(a) may result in jugular vein distention.

(b) is caused by blood in the pericardial sac (outside the heart) exerting pressure on the heart.

(c) will cause a falling systolic blood pressure and a rising diastolic blood pressure.

(d) All of the above.

(e) None of the above.

110. Cardiac tamponade

(a) may result in jugular vein distention.

(b) is caused by blood in the pericardial sac (outside the heart) exerting pressure on the heart.

(c) will cause a falling systolic blood pressure and a rising diastolic blood pressure.

(d) All of the above.

(e) None of the above.

111. Tension pneumothorax

(a) may result in jugular vein distention.

(b) is caused by blood in the pericardial sac (outside the heart) exerting pressure on the heart.

(c) will cause a falling systolic blood pressure and a rising diastolic blood pressure.

(d) All of the above.

(e) None of the above.

112. The esophagus is
    (a) a distal portion of the small intestines.
    (b) a tube extending from the oropharynx to the stomach.
    (c) a proximal portion of the large intestines.
    (d) the voice box.
    (e) the stomach.

113. The solid organs in the abdomen include the
    (a) gallbladder, spleen, pancreas, and urinary bladder.
    (b) heart, lungs, pancreas, and liver.
    (c) urinary bladder, spleen, liver, and intestines.
    (d) spleen, liver, pancreas, and kidneys.
    (e) stomach, intestines, and gallbladder.

114. The hollow abdominal organs include the
    (a) gallbladder, spleen, pancreas, and urinary bladder.
    (b) heart, lungs, pancreas, and liver.
    (c) urinary bladder, spleen, liver, and intestines.
    (d) spleen, liver, pancreas, and kidneys.
    (e) stomach, intestines, and gallbladder.

115. Although the kidneys are frequently considered to be abdominal organs, they are actually located in the
    (a) chest cavity.
    (b) back cavity.
    (c) retroperitoneal cavity.
    (d) peritoneal cavity.
    (e) pelvic cavity.

116. Although the urinary bladder is frequently considered to be an abdominal organ, it is actually located in the
    (a) chest cavity.
    (b) back cavity.
    (c) retroperitoneal cavity.
    (d) peritoneal cavity.
    (e) pelvic cavity.

117. The pancreas
    (a) is considered part of the digestive system.
    (b) is considered part of the urinary system.
    (c) is considered part of the reproductive system.
    (d) All of the above.
    (e) None of the above.

118. The prostate gland
    (a) is considered part of the digestive system.
    (b) is considered part of the urinary system.
    (c) is considered part of the reproductive system.
    (d) All of the above.
    (e) None of the above.

119. The liver
    (a) is considered part of the digestive system.
    (b) is considered part of the urinary system.
    (c) is considered part of the reproductive system.
    (d) All of the above.
    (e) None of the above.

120. The kidneys
    (a) are considered part of the digestive system.
    (b) are considered part of the urinary system.
    (c) are considered part of the reproductive system.
    (d) All of the above.
    (e) None of the above.

121. The seminal vesicles
    (a) are considered part of the digestive system.
    (b) are considered part of the urinary system.
    (c) are considered part of the reproductive system.
    (d) All of the above.
    (e) None of the above.

122. The adrenal glands
    (a) are considered part of the digestive system.
    (b) are considered part of the urinary system.
    (c) are considered part of the reproductive system.
    (d) All of the above.
    (e) None of the above.

123. The gallbladder and bile ducts
    (a) are considered part of the digestive system.
    (b) are considered part of the urinary system.
    (c) are considered part of the reproductive system.
    (d) All of the above.
    (e) None of the above.

124. The ureters
- (a) are considered part of the digestive system.
- (b) are considered part of the urinary system.
- (c) are considered part of the reproductive system.
- (d) All of the above.
- (e) None of the above.

125. The spleen
- (a) is considered part of the digestive system.
- (b) is considered part of the urinary system.
- (c) is considered part of the reproductive system.
- (d) All of the above.
- (e) None of the above.

126. The appendix
- (a) is considered part of the digestive system.
- (b) is considered part of the urinary system.
- (c) is considered part of the reproductive system.
- (d) All of the above.
- (e) None of the above.

127. The spleen
- (a) can be ruptured as a result of blunt trauma to the right lower quadrant of the abdomen.
- (b) produces a substance called "chyme," which assists in digestion of food.
- (c) assists in absorption of nutrients by storing blood.
- (d) functions to remove old blood cells and to store blood.
- (e) produces a substance called peptic acid, which assists in digestion of food.

128. The peritoneum is
- (a) the division between the abdominal cavity and the retroperitoneal space.
- (b) a lining that covers the abdominal organs.
- (c) the lining of the abdominal cavity.
- (d) All of the above.
- (e) None of the above.

129. Peritonitis is an inflammation of
- (a) the division between the abdominal cavity and the retroperitoneal space.
- (b) a lining that covers the abdominal organs.

(c) the lining of the abdominal cavity.

(d) All of the above.

(e) None of the above.

130. Peritonitis can be caused by all of the following except

(a) infection from an open abdominal wound.

(b) free blood in the abdomen.

(c) digestive enzymes loose in the abdomen.

(d) bowel contents loose in the abdomen.

(e) pneumonia with a productive cough.

131. A projectile object (such as a bullet)

(a) creates a direct line of injury from entrance to exit wound.

(b) can deflect and shatter within the body, causing extensive hidden damage.

(c) is usually dense enough to remain intact.

(d) causes a more severe injury when it has both an entrance and an exit wound.

(e) creates a larger entry wound than exit wound because the force of initial impact is absorbed by the body tissues.

132. Signs and symptoms of severe abdominal injury include all of the following except

(a) blood in the urine.

(b) coffee-ground vomitus.

(c) bradycardia and hypotension.

(d) tachypnea and shallow breathing.

(e) the patient lying very still, usually with the legs drawn up.

133. Emergency care of abdominal injuries includes all of the following except

(a) anticipate shock and work to prevent it.

(b) constantly monitor and evaluate the vital signs.

(c) be alert for vomitus; have suction ready.

(d) do not remove penetrating objects; surround them with an occlusive dressing and stabilize them in place with bulky dressings.

(e) gently return protruding organs to their protective cavity and cover with a sterile occlusive dressing.

134. The body structures and organs found in the pelvic cavity include
- (a) the adrenal glands, the appendix, the urinary bladder, and the spleen.
- (b) the kidneys, the ureters, the urinary bladder, and the urethra.
- (c) the internal genitalia, the transverse colon, and the inferior vena cava.
- (d) the femoral artery, the femoral vein, and the prostate and adrenal glands.
- (e) the femoral arteries and veins, the urinary bladder, the rectum, and internal genitalia.

135. Which of the following statements regarding injuries to the external male genitalia is true?
- (a) As with injuries to other body parts, there may be bruises, lacerations, penetrating objects, and avulsions.
- (b) Blood in the urethra should be considered a sign of pelvic fracture.
- (c) Blood in the urine should be considered a sign of a urinary system problem.
- (d) All of the above are true.
- (e) None of the above is true.

136. The penis
- (a) produces male hormone and sperm cells.
- (b) produces fluids that combine with sperm to create semen.
- (c) stores semen.
- (d) surrounds the testes.
- (e) contains the urethra.

137. The scrotum
- (a) produces male hormone and sperm cells.
- (b) produces fluids that combine with sperm to create semen.
- (c) stores semen.
- (d) surrounds the testes.
- (e) contains the urethra.

138. The prostate gland
- (a) produces male hormone and sperm cells.
- (b) produces fluids that combine with sperm to create semen.

    (c)   stores semen.
    (d)   surrounds the testes.
    (e)   contains the urethra.

139. The testicles
    (a)   produce male hormone and sperm cells.
    (b)   produce fluids that combine with sperm to create semen.
    (c)   store semen.
    (d)   surround the testes.
    (e)   contain the urethra.

140. The seminal vesicles
    (a)   produce male hormone and sperm cells.
    (b)   produce fluids that combine with sperm to create semen.
    (c)   store semen.
    (d)   surround the testes.
    (e)   contain the urethra.

141. The vagina
    (a)   produces female hormones and eggs.
    (b)   is the female external genitalia.
    (c)   is the location of a normal pregnancy.
    (d)   is also called the birth canal.
    (e)   is the location of most ectopic pregnancies.

142. The vulva
    (a)   produces female hormones and eggs.
    (b)   is the female external genitalia.
    (c)   is the location of a normal pregnancy.
    (d)   is also called the birth canal.
    (e)   is the location of most ectopic pregnancies.

143. The ovaries
    (a)   produce female hormones and eggs.
    (b)   are the female external genitalia.
    (c)   are the location of a normal pregnancy.
    (d)   are also called the birth canal.
    (e)   are the location of most ectopic pregnancies.

144. The fallopian tubes
   (a) produce female hormones and eggs.
   (b) are the female external genitalia.
   (c) are the location of a normal pregnancy.
   (d) are also called the birth canal.
   (e) are the location of most ectopic pregnancies.

145. The uterus
   (a) produces female hormones and eggs.
   (b) is the female external genitalia.
   (c) is the location of a normal pregnancy.
   (d) is also called the birth canal.
   (e) is the location of most ectopic pregnancies.

146. The condition commonly known as a hernia occurs when
   (a) an infection causes a bowel obstruction.
   (b) a bowel obstruction becomes inflamed.
   (c) a testicle becomes twisted and swollen.
   (d) a male reaches the age of 40 years old.
   (e) a part of the intestine bulges through a defect in the diaphragm or abdominal wall.

147. The area located between the external genitalia and the anus is called the
   (a) perineum.
   (b) cervix.
   (c) vagina.
   (d) uterus.
   (e) vulva.

148. The muscular, elastic organ that contains the developing baby is called the
   (a) perineum.
   (b) cervix.
   (c) vagina.
   (d) uterus.
   (e) vulva.

149. All of the following items belong in a standard obstetrical kit except
   (a) sterile gloves, 4 X 4 gauze pads, sanitary napkins.
   (b) a sterile scalpel.
   (c) one or more plastic bags.
   (d) two or more sterile, sharp hemostats.
   (e) an infant suction device.

150. When the baby is developing within the womb it is called

    (a) an amniotic sac.
    (b) an embryonic sac.
    (c) a fetus.
    (d) an infant.
    (e) a placenta.

151. The structure that is found at the distal end of the womb, before the birth canal, is called the

    (a) perineum.
    (b) cervix.
    (c) vagina.
    (d) uterus.
    (e) vulva.

152. The umbilical cord connects the developing baby to the

    (a) amniotic sac.
    (b) embryonic sac.
    (c) fetus.
    (d) infant.
    (e) placenta.

153. The developing baby is contained within the

    (a) amniotic sac.
    (b) embryonic sac.
    (c) fetus.
    (d) infant.
    (e) placenta.

154. Which of the following statements regarding the developing baby is true?

    (a) Oxygen and carbon dioxide are constantly being exchanged within the fluid that surrounds the baby in the sac.
    (b) The bag of waters is attached to the walls of the womb to prevent rupture during trauma.
    (c) The mother's blood flows through the placenta and circulates within the fetus, distributing nutrients and removing wastes. It then passes back through the placenta to the mother's system, where the wastes are disposed of and more nutrients obtained.
    (d) All of the above are true.
    (e) None of the above is true.

155. Full dilation of the cervix signifies
  (a) the beginning of the fourth stage of labor.
  (b) the end of the second stage of labor.
  (c) the end of the first stage of labor.
  (d) the beginning of the first stage of labor.
  (e) the end of the third stage of labor.

156. The birth of the baby signifies
  (a) the beginning of the fourth stage of labor.
  (b) the end of the second stage of labor.
  (c) the end of the first stage of labor.
  (d) the beginning of the first stage of labor.
  (e) the end of the third stage of labor.

157. The beginning of regular contractions signifies
  (a) the beginning of the fourth stage of labor.
  (b) the end of the second stage of labor.
  (c) the end of the first stage of labor.
  (d) the beginning of the first stage of labor.
  (e) the end of the third stage of labor.

158. The delivery of the afterbirth signifies
  (a) the beginning of the fourth stage of labor.
  (b) the end of the second stage of labor.
  (c) the end of the first stage of labor.
  (d) the beginning of the first stage of labor.
  (e) the end of the third stage of labor.

159. As delivery begins, when the baby's head is the first part to be seen it is called a
  (a) cephalic presentation.
  (b) breech presentation.
  (c) occipital presentation.
  (d) head presentation.
  (e) posterior presentation.

160. As delivery begins, when the baby's bottom is the first part to be seen it is called a
  (a) cephalic presentation.
  (b) breech presentation.
  (c) occipital presentation.
  (d) head presentation.
  (e) posterior presentation.

161. When the baby's head can be seen pushing at the opening of the birth canal, it is called

    (a) crowing.
    (b) dilation.
    (c) crowning.
    (d) breeching.
    (e) bearing down.

162. When the baby's bottom can be seen pushing at the opening of the birth canal, it is called

    (a) crowing.
    (b) dilation.
    (c) crowning.
    (d) breeching.
    (e) bearing down.

163. When the cervix expands to allow passage of the baby, it is called

    (a) crowing.
    (b) dilation.
    (c) crowning.
    (d) breeching.
    (e) bearing down.

164. "Bloody show" is defined as

    (a) an active bleeding that accompanies the first stage of labor.
    (b) an active bleeding that accompanies the second stage of labor.
    (c) an active bleeding that accompanies the third stage of labor.
    (d) a discharge of watery mucous that contains a small amount of blood and indicates that actual labor is in progress.
    (e) a discharge of mucous and blood, indicating that birth will rapidly occur.

165. The answer to the question, "How far apart are your contractions?" is the time from

    (a) the start of a contraction to its end, when the womb
        relaxes.

    (b) the end of one contraction to the beginning of the next
        contraction.

    (c) when the mother feels like pushing to when she feels like
        panting.

    (d) the end of one contraction to the end of the next
        contraction.

    (e) the start of one contraction to the start of the next
        contraction.

166. The answer to the question, "How long do your contractions
last?" is the time from

    (a) the start of a contraction to its end, when the womb
        relaxes.

    (b) the end of one contraction to the beginning of the next
        contraction.

    (c) when the mother feels like pushing to when she feels like
        panting.

    (d) the end of one contraction to the end of the next
        contraction.

    (e) the start of one contraction to the start of the next
        contraction.

167. Which of the following statements regarding false labor
pains is false? False labor pains are

    (a) generally limited to the lower abdomen with little to no
        back involvement.

    (b) caused by the changes that occur in the size and shape
        of the womb, usually during the last month of
        pregnancy.

    (c) easily mistaken for true labor pains because of their
        regular pattern of contraction.

    (d) All of the above are false.

    (e) None of the above is false.

168. It is important to ask a mother if this is her first pregnancy
because

    (a) documentation of abortions, miscarriages, and live births
        is a legal record.

    (b) first pregnancies frequently deliver rapidly.

(c) each subsequent pregnancy will occur in the same manner as the first.

(d) All of the above.

(e) None of the above.

169. When the mother insists on using the toilet to move her bowels, the EMT should

    (a) have a female assist her to the bathroom.

    (b) refuse to allow her to do so and transport her to the hospital immediately.

    (c) find a basin or tub that can be used as a bed pan.

    (d) prepare for delivery.

    (e) boil water.

170. Your patient is 23 years old and its her first pregnancy. She denies the need to bear down but has been having contractions for the past 2 hours and they are now 5 minutes apart. She called 911 because her bag of waters just broke. You can see no presenting part pushing at the birth canal opening. You should

    (a) prepare for a rapid delivery.

    (b) transport her to the hospital.

    (c) wait on scene for no more than 20 minutes for birth to occur.

    (d) wait on scene for 30 minutes to accurately time her contractions.

    (e) prepare for an abnormal delivery.

171. Supine hypotensive syndrome is defined as

    (a) low blood pressure caused by the weight of the developing baby preventing return of blood to the heart.

    (b) high blood pressure caused by the weight of the developing baby preventing blood from leaving the heart.

    (c) dizziness that goes away when the patient lies down.

    (d) low blood pressure that occurs when the baby is about to deliver.

    (e) high blood pressure that occurs when the baby is about to deliver.

172. If delivery is going to take place in an automobile

   (a) move the mother to the ambulance first.
   (b) move the mother to the back seat for additional room to work in.
   (c) have the mother put both feet up on the dash or the back of the front seat.
   (d) have the mother place one foot on the floor board.
   (e) have the mother place both feet on the floor board.

173. When the baby's head appears, place the fingers of your gloved hand

   (a) on the perineum and push gently to assist in the delivery.
   (b) on the baby's head and exert very gentle pressure to prevent an explosive delivery.
   (c) near the area where the head is seen so that the baby will emerge into your hands (and not be dropped!).
   (d) All of the above.
   (e) None of the above.

174. If the bag of waters does not break

   (a) use your fingers to pinch and puncture the sac; then push the sac away from the baby's nose and mouth for suctioning.
   (b) continue with the delivery; the sac will break on its own once the baby is completely delivered.
   (c) use a scalpel to carefully open the sac before the baby takes its first breath.
   (d) leave the sac alone unless the baby appears to be breathing.
   (e) delay further delivery and transport immediately (a cesarean section will be required).

175. When the head emerges, if the umbilical cord is wrapped around the baby's neck and cannot be gently loosened

   (a) continue with the delivery; the cord will unwind as the baby is completely delivered.
   (b) delay further delivery and transport immediately (a cesarean section will be required).
   (c) clamp or tie the cord in two places and cut the cord between the clamps/ties.
   (d) forcefully pull the cord over the baby's head before the baby is strangled.
   (e) do not delay for clamping or tying; cut the cord and remove it before the baby is strangled.

176. Suction the baby's airway
    (a) only after the baby is safely delivered.
    (b) only after the baby has started making efforts to breathe (to do so earlier may cause injury).
    (c) only after the umbilical cord has been cut.
    (d) only after the baby is safely in its mother's arms.
    (e) as soon as the head has delivered.

177. When a newborn's airway is suctioned,
    (a) the mouth is to be suctioned before the nose.
    (b) the nose is to be suctioned before the mouth.
    (c) either the nose or mouth can be suctioned first.
    (d) the suction tip is to be inserted as far as the EMT can reach to elicit a gag reflex.
    (e) the suction tip is to be deeply inserted into the infant's nostrils to ensure removal of all fluids.

178. Assessment of the newborn should be performed
    (a) in the ambulance, on the way to the hospital.
    (b) at 1 and 5 minutes after birth.
    (c) at 1 and 5 minutes after the birth of the placenta.
    (d) at 5 and 10 minutes after the birth of the placenta.
    (e) at 7 and 13 minutes after birth.

179. When the APGAR scoring system is used to assess the newborn, the two "A"s stand for
    (a) appearance (skin color) and absent respirations (breathing).
    (b) activity (extremity movement) and altered mentation (level of consciousness).
    (c) appearance (skin color) and activity (extremity movement).
    (d) appearance (skin color) and activity (heart rate).
    (e) activity (grimace) and appearance (extremity movement).

180. When the APGAR scoring system is used to assess the newborn, the "P" stands for
    (a) pulse (heart rate).
    (b) pupils (equal or unequal).
    (c) pink (skin color).
    (d) pallor (skin color).
    (e) purple (cyanosis).

181. When the APGAR scoring system is used to assess the newborn, the "G" stands for

    (a) gasping (poor respiratory effort).
    (b) gurgling (indications of aspiration).
    (c) gross deformity (abnormal infant).
    (d) grimace (irritability/crying).
    (e) groaning (poor ability to cry).

182. When the APGAR scoring system is used to assess the newborn, the "R" stands for

    (a) rigor (stillborn infant).
    (b) rapid (heart rate or respiratory rate).
    (c) rate (of pulse or respirations).
    (d) respirations (rate and effort of respiration).
    (e) robust (health, crying infant).

183. As soon as the baby is born, keep it

    (a) on its side with the head elevated to allow for adequate suction of its mouth and nose.
    (b) stimulated by exposure to room temperature air.
    (c) on its back with the head slightly lower than its body to allow for adequate drainage of the airway.
    (d) wrapped in a warm blanket and on its side with the head elevated.
    (e) wrapped in a warm blanket and on its side with the head slightly lower to allow for drainage and suction of fluids.

184. Washing of the newborn is done

    (a) immediately after birth to avoid infection.
    (b) by the mother, as she nurses the infant en route to the hospital.
    (c) only after arrival at the hospital.
    (d) to stimulate the baby to breathe.
    (e) after the umbilical cord has been cut.

185. The umbilical cord is

    (a) first clamped off about 2 to 3 inches away from the baby.
    (b) to be cut when the newborn's APGAR score is 10.
    (c) not to be clamped or cut if the infant is not breathing unless CPR is required.
    (d) cut after the placenta delivers.
    (e) cut only after the child has begun nursing to replace fluids.

186. Given the fact that delivery of the placenta is accompanied by bleeding, the EMT should
  (a) gently insert a rolled sanitary napkin in the vagina.
  (b) expect excessive blood loss which will rarely lead to shock.
  (c) gently massage the mother's abdomen to assist in uterine contraction.
  (d) All of the above.
  (e) None of the above.

187. Afterbirth is
  (a) the period of time following a delivery.
  (b) the fourth stage of delivery.
  (c) the improper fertilization of the egg.
  (d) a severe complication of a delivery that results in convulsions and shock.
  (e) the placenta, sac membranes, and tissues from the lining of the uterus that are delivered after the birth of the baby.

188. Which of the following statements regarding delivery of the placenta is true?
  (a) It is not necessary to wait for the delivery of the placenta.
  (b) Save all portions of the placenta in a plastic bag and transport it to the hospital with mother and baby.
  (c) Do not delay transport longer than 20 minutes for the delivery of the placenta.
  (d) All of the above are true.
  (e) None of the above is true.

189. External massage of the uterus
  (a) is an invasion of privacy, and the EMT can be charged with assault and battery if it is performed.
  (b) is necessary only if excessive bleeding has occurred.
  (c) will encourage contraction of the uterus to aid in control of bleeding.
  (d) is necessary only if the mother will not breast-feed the baby.
  (e) may cause aspiration or choking and therefore should not be allowed in the ambulance.

190. External massage of the breasts
- (a) is an invasion of privacy, and the EMT can be charged with assault and battery if it is performed.
- (b) is necessary only if excessive bleeding has occurred.
- (c) will encourage contraction of the uterus to aid in control of bleeding.
- (d) is necessary only if the mother will not breast-feed the baby.
- (e) may cause aspiration or choking and therefore should not be allowed in the ambulance.

191. Encouraging the mother to nurse the baby
- (a) is an invasion of privacy, and the EMT can be charged with assault and battery if it is performed.
- (b) is necessary only if excessive bleeding has occurred.
- (c) will encourage contraction of the uterus to aid in control of bleeding.
- (d) is necessary only if the mother will not breast-feed the baby.
- (e) may cause aspiration or choking and therefore should not be allowed in the ambulance.

192. Mothers at high risk of developing complications during delivery are those who
- (a) are over 35 years of age or have had 5 or more previous pregnancies.
- (b) have had twins in the past.
- (c) have had cesarean sections in the past.
- (d) All of the above.
- (e) None of the above.

193. The acceptable forms of stimulating a newborn to breathe are
- (a) inverting the infant to facilitate fluid drainage from the airway and gently but briskly spank the infant's bottom.
- (b) vigorous but gentle rubbing of the infant's back with a dry cloth. If unsuccessful, snap your fingers against the soles of the infant's feet.
- (c) lightly sprinking cool water onto the baby's back and then vigorously drying the back with a soft cloth.
- (d) All of the above.
- (e) None of the above.

194. CPR is required for a newborn when
  (a) respirations are absent.
  (b) the baby is breathing but has a pulse rate less than 80 per minute.
  (c) the pulse is absent.
  (d) Answers (a) and (c) only.
  (e) Answers (a), (b), and (c).

195. Which of the following statements regarding prehospital delivery of a baby is true?
  (a) The EMTs should notify the dispatcher that they are delivering a baby at home and may be out of service for more than an hour.
  (b) The EMTs should notify the dispatcher that they are delivering a baby at home and will be on scene for no more than one hour.
  (c) After 20 minutes of contractions every 2 to 3 minutes, transport the patient to the hospital.
  (d) After 20 minutes of contractions every 2 to 3 minutes, notify the dispatcher that you are safe and will be on scene longer than expected.
  (e) After 10 minutes of contractions every 2 to 3 minutes, transport the patient to the hospital.

196. In the event of excessive prebirth bleeding
  (a) apply MAST trousers and inflate the legs only.
  (b) place the patient on her left side, treat for shock, and transport her to the hospital.
  (c) gently insert a rolled sanitary napkin in the vagina, turn the patient onto her left side, and wait for the bleeding to stop before proceeding with the delivery.
  (d) gently massage the mother's abdomen to assist in uterine contraction.
  (e) relax; excessive bleeding is a common occurence in all deliveries and you should proceed as normal.

197. Which of the following statements regarding placenta previa is false?
  (a) It occurs when all or some of the placenta is between the baby and the cervix.
  (b) It presents with painless vaginal bleeding, usually late in the pregnancy.
  (c) It will not allow for normal delivery of the baby.
  (d) It is often not accompanied by external bleeding and is usually very painful.
  (e) It can result in fetal death.

198. Which of the following statements regarding abruptio placentae is false?

    (a) It is a complete or partial separation of the placenta from the wall of the womb.

    (b) It presents with painless vaginal bleeding, usually late in the pregnancy.

    (c) It is usually caused by deceleration forces or direct trauma.

    (d) It is often not accompanied by external bleeding and is usually extremely painful.

    (e) It may produce the onset of premature labor.

199. Toxemia of pregnancy

    (a) can be recognized when the patient has extreme swelling of the face and hands and is hypertensive.

    (b) is present when the patient is an epileptic.

    (c) can be recognized when the patient has swollen feet and is hypotensive.

    (d) is present when the patient complains of headache and abdominal pain.

    (e) is an abdominal infection that frequently results in seizures.

200. Eclampsia can be recognized when the pregnant patient

    (a) has extreme swelling of the face and hands.

    (b) when the patient complains of headache and is hypertensive.

    (c) is an epileptic.

    (d) All of the above.

    (e) None of the above.

201. Treatment for toxemia of pregnancy includes all of the following except

    (a) place the mother on her left side.

    (b) administer high-flow oxygen.

    (c) transport gently, but with lights and sirens to accomplish arrival at the hospital before the onset of seizures.

    (d) be prepared to provide suction for vomitus.

    (e) have the obstetric kit ready in case of delivery.

202. Which of the following statements regarding ectopic pregnancy is false?

    (a) An ectopic pregnancy is one in which implantation of the fertilized egg occurs outside the womb.

    (b) Any woman of childbearing age with acute abdominal pain or unexplained shock must be considered to have a possible ectopic pregnancy.

    (c) Ectopic pregnancies present with gross vaginal bleeding.

    (d) An ectopic pregnancy is a life-threatening emergency.

    (e) An ectopic pregnancy occurs in the early stages of a pregnancy.

203. Which of the following statements regarding treatment of the pregnant trauma patient is false?

    (a) If the mechanism of injury suggests spinal injury, apply a cervical collar, secure her to a long backboard, and elevate the right side of the backboard.

    (b) Administer oxygen only by nasal cannula, as high-flow oxygen will cause fetal injury.

    (c) Despite the patient's denial of injury, all pregnant trauma patients should be transported to the hospital.

    (d) All of the above are false.

    (e) None of the above is false.

204. Miscarriage

    (a) is an outdated term and should be called a "spontaneous abortion" instead.

    (b) is an induced abortion unless it happens very early in the pregnancy (when it might be a normal loss).

    (c) requires questioning to determine whether it was spontaneous or induced, because it is the duty of the EMT to report all abortions to law enforcement agencies.

    (d) All of the above.

    (e) None of the above.

205. A ruptured uterus

    (a) frequently occurs spontaneously and is a life-threatening emergency.

    (b) can occur during labor or because of trauma.

    (c) causes extreme pain and will present with excessive external bleeding.

    (d) All of the above.

    (e) None of the above.

206. A limb presentation is when
  (a) the baby appears both feet first during delivery.
  (b) the baby appears face first during delivery.
  (c) the umbilical cord appears first during delivery.
  (d) All of the above.
  (e) None of the above.

207. The baby cannot be delivered in the field if
  (a) the baby appears both feet first during delivery.
  (b) the baby appears face first during delivery.
  (c) the umbilical cord appears first during delivery.
  (d) All of the above.
  (e) None of the above.

208. Which of the following statements regarding abnormal deliveries is false?
  (a) If a prolapsed cord becomes cold, the oxygen supply to the unborn infant will be stopped and the infant will die.
  (b) The insertion of a gloved hand into the mother's vagina may be necessary to gently push a baby's head off of a prolapsed cord.
  (c) The insertion of a gloved hand into the mother's vagina may be necessary to gently replace a single-limb presentation.
  (d) The insertion of a gloved hand into the mother's vagina may be necessary to provide an airway for the breech-birth baby whose head will not deliver.
  (e) If both feet present first, the baby may still be delivered in the field.

209. When a delivery becomes a multiple-birth situation, it is important to
  (a) be on your way to the hospital before the second or third baby delivers.
  (b) suction and warm one infant before delivering the next.
  (c) wait for delivery of the first baby's placenta before allowing the next baby to deliver.
  (d) All of the above.
  (e) None of the above.

210. When caring for the premature newborn, the EMT must
  (a) prevent heat loss by thoroughly drying the baby and wrapping it in a foil-lined blanket.
  (b) provide oxygenation and maintain a clear airway with suctioning.

(c) protect the baby from external sources of contamination.

(d) All of the above.

(e) None of the above.

211. Typically the sources of a radiation burn are

(a) AC/DC currents and lightning.

(b) ultraviolet light and nuclear agents.

(c) nuclear agents only.

(d) lightning only.

(e) chemicals (acids, bases, corrosives).

212. As opposed to falls or trauma that may occur after the burn, fractures and burns can be directly caused by

(a) AC/DC currents and lightning.

(b) ultraviolet light and nuclear agents.

(c) nuclear agents only.

(d) lightning only.

(e) chemicals (acids, bases, corrosives).

213. A partial-thickness burn is also called

(a) a first-degree burn.

(b) a second-degree burn.

(c) a third-degree burn.

(d) Both answers (a) and (b).

(e) Both answers (b) and (c).

214. Blisters are associated with

(a) a first-degree burn.

(b) a second-degree burn.

(c) a third-degree burn.

(d) Both answers (a) and (b).

(e) Both answers (b) and (c).

215. Loss of sensation due to a destruction of nerve endings is associated with

(a) a first-degree burn.

(b) a second-degree burn.

(c) a third-degree burn.

(d) Both answers (a) and (b).

(e) Both answers (b) and (c).

216. Severe pain may be associated with all areas of

    (a) a first-degree burn.

    (b) a second-degree burn.

    (c) a third-degree burn.

    (d) Both answers (a) and (b).

    (e) Both answers (b) and (c).

217. A full-thickness burn is also called

    (a) a first-degree burn.

    (b) a second-degree burn.

    (c) a third-degree burn.

    (d) Both answers (a) and (b).

    (e) Both answers (b) and (c).

218. Charred black and dry white areas are associated with

    (a) a first-degree burn.

    (b) a second-degree burn.

    (c) a third-degree burn.

    (d) Both answers (a) and (b).

    (e) Both answers (b) and (c).

219. The sun can cause

    (a) a first-degree burn.

    (b) a second-degree burn.

    (c) a third-degree burn.

    (d) Both answers (a) and (b).

    (e) Both answers (b) and (c)

220. Which of the following statements regarding circumferential burns is true?

    (a) A circumferential burn is one that completely encircles the body or extremity.

    (b) A circumferential burn can obstruct circulation to the unburned areas beyond the burn.

    (c) A circumferential burn can obstruct normal function of an area despite the absence of injury beneath the burn.

    (d) All of the above are true.

    (e) None of the above is true.

221. An example of a critical burn is

    (a) a burn involving the airway.

    (b) a first-degree burn involving 50 percent of the body surface.

(c) a second-degree burn involving 15 percent of the body surface.
(d) any third-degree burn.
(e) a circumferential burn.

222. What percentage of body surface is affected if a child is burned on the front and back of both legs?
  (a) 14 percent.
  (b) 18 percent.
  (c) 27 percent.
  (d) 28 percent.
  (e) 50 percent.

223. What percentage of body surface is affected if an adult is burned on the back of both legs and lower torso?
  (a) 14 percent.
  (b) 18 percent.
  (c) 27 percent.
  (d) 28 percent.
  (e) 50 percent.

224. If a patient with multiple first-degree burns presents in a hypotensive state, the EMT should
  (a) classify the extent of the burn as being full thickness.
  (b) treat with high-flow oxygen.
  (c) suspect underlying medical problems or trauma.
  (d) Both answers (a) and (b).
  (e) Both answers (b) and (c).

225. When treating a victim of burns, the EMT should never apply
  (a) antiseptic spray.
  (b) an antibiotic burn cream.
  (c) ice.
  (d) Both answers (a) and (b).
  (e) Any of the above.

226. The EMT's first priority in treating a burn patient is to
  (a) assess the airway.
  (b) eliminate the source of the burn.
  (c) determine the depth and percentage of the burn.
  (d) determine the mechanism of injury.
  (e) perform a complete primary survey.

227. Which of the following statements regarding care for chemical burns is false?

    (a) Most chemical burns should be throughly irrigated with water and then covered with a dry sheet.

    (b) Dry lime should be brushed from the skin and clothing prior to irrigation.

    (c) Hot wax or tar must be pulled or scraped off the body's surface in the field to effectively stop the burning process.

    (d) Carbolic acid must be initially washed from unbroken skin with alcohol, followed by water washing.

    (e) Both answers (c) and (d) are false.

228. Smoke inhalation

    (a) can injure the airway and cause respiratory arrest.

    (b) is a frequent minor injury and requires little treatment beyond nasal cannula oxygen administration.

    (c) is serious only if the patient was in an enclosed, smoke-filled place for more than 10 minutes.

    (d) All of the above.

    (e) None of the above.

229. The correct treatment for chemical burns to the eyes is to

    (a) provide flushing with copious amounts of water for at least 20 minutes.

    (b) first neutralize the chemical with vinegar, and then flush with water.

    (c) first neutralize the chemical with baking soda, and then flush with water.

    (d) allow the patient's tears to maintain eye moisture.

    (e) use only sterile water when irrigating the eyes.

230. Which of the following statements regarding electrical burns is false?

    (a) If a power line is charged and in contact with a vehicle, the occupants are safe unless fire or explosion occurs.

    (b) The major problem with electrical burns is respiratory and cardiac arrest.

    (c) The burn commonly enters in one place but leaves the body in another, causing two external burns only.

    (d) All of the above are false.

    (e) None of the above is false.

231. Which of the following statements regarding radiation burns is true?

    (a) Alpha and beta particles are the most penetrating and dangerous.

    (b) Gamma rays are dangerous only if the particles they irradiate are swallowed or inhaled.

    (c) X-ray machines do not irradiate body cells.

    (d) All of the above are true.

    (e) None of the above is true.

232. Hazardous materials incidents

    (a) are easy to deal with once the substance is identified.

    (b) are off-limits to untrained EMTs even when the appropriate safety equipment is available.

    (c) will usually have a distinctive odor that will warn the EMT of their presence.

    (d) All of the above.

    (e) None of the above.

233. Treatment for radiation burns

    (a) is the same as treatment for electrical burns.

    (b) requires special procedures and showers.

    (c) is the same as treatment for chemical burns.

    (d) should be delayed until a Geiger counter is present.

    (e) is the same as treatment for thermal burns.

234. All of the following represent effective and responsible methods of communication with patients except

    (a) keeping eye contact unless the patient appears threatened by it.

    (b) using terms that can be understood.

    (c) answering questions honestly, unless you anticipate the patient to respond adversely.

    (d) properly identifying yourself.

    (e) being direct and not giving the patient "false hope."

235. A patient's normal response to terminal illness may include all of the following except

    (a) hostility and anger.

    (b) acceptance.

    (c) bargaining.

    (d) denial and depression.

    (e) mental illness.

236. A family's normal response to the death of a loved one long known to have a terminal illness includes all of the following except

    (a) hostility and anger.
    (b) acceptance.
    (c) bargaining.
    (d) denial and depression.
    (e) mental illness.

237. Your patient is combative, hostile, and very confused. He refuses to let you near him. He is 20 years old and has no obvious trauma. His skin is warm, dry, and pink. There is no odor of alcohol on his breath. Which of the following statements regarding your patient is true?

    (a) As long as he has not commited a crime, the police will not be able to assist you.
    (b) Despite the fact that he is an adult, his confused state enables you to have the police initiate protective custody arrest or a mental health hold; therefore enabling you to apply restraints and provide care.
    (c) Although you suspect hidden closed head injury, diabetes, or psychiatric disorder, you cannot treat him as long as he refuses. Your only course of action is to wait until he becomes unresponsive.
    (d) Since there is no sign of trauma and his skin is warm, dry, and pink (ruling out diabetes), you may assume that the patient is either on drugs or a psych-case and therefore does not need an ambulance.
    (e) If a patient threatens you with harm, simply leave the scene. If his behavior continues, someone else will call the police and it will become their problem—not yours.

238. Standard restraint procedures include all of the following except

    (a) use only restraints that will not inflict injury.
    (b) plastic disposable restraints are the most humane and effective.
    (c) once the patient is restrained, do not remove the restraints until after arrival at the ER.
    (d) use leather or layered gauze bandage restraints.
    (e) restrain combative patients only in the presence of police officers.

239. When providing care for a patient who has expressed suicidal ideation, it is vitally important to remember
    (a) to ask about a plan; the patient who actually has a plan for suicide is in more immediate danger.
    (b) that some psychiatric medicines (especially those for depression) provide lethal means of overdose.
    (c) the ABCs.
    (d) that "suicidal" ideation can easily be refocused and become "homicidal" ideation.
    (e) to call in a mental health professional; the EMT is poorly equipped to deal with suicidal emergencies.

240. When dealing with a victim of rape, the EMT should
    (a) avoid destruction of evidence by not examining the patient; provide emotional support and transport the patient without lights and sirens.
    (b) obtain as much information as possible to aid in the police investigation; patients frequently forget important aspects of the crime after they have been at the hospital for hours.
    (c) provide emotional support while concentrating on medical care only.
    (d) Answers (a) and (b) only.
    (e) All of the above.

241. Indications of EMT stress syndrome include all of the following except
    (a) alcohol or drug abuse.
    (b) excessive fatigue, frequent nightmares, insomnia.
    (c) chronic irritability and inability to concentrate.
    (d) frequent muscle aches, headaches, nausea.
    (e) seeking professional help.

242. The ways to prevent or reduce the development of stress syndrome include
    (a) seeking peer support, taking extra time off, considering the reasons you became an EMT.
    (b) taking time off or quitting the service you work for.
    (c) developing the ability to ignore the problems that cause you distress.
    (d) taking psychiatric medications.
    (e) forcing yourself to "relive" distressful calls until you become accustomed to them.

243. Peristalsis is defined as

   (a) an infection of the esophagus or intestines frequently causing bowel obstruction.

   (b) an inflammation of the intestines frequently causing bowel obstruction.

   (c) a wavelike motion that occurs in hollow tubes of the body, causing movement of the contents from one place to another.

   (d) All of the above.

   (e) None of the above.

244. The soft spots between the cranial bones of the newborn's skull are called

   (a) follicles.

   (b) fontanels.

   (c) fountains.

   (d) phalanxes.

   (e) phobias.

245. The mediastinum

   (a) contains the heart, large blood vessels, and parts of the trachea and esophagus.

   (b) surrounds the heart and contains a small amount of fluid that prevents friction as the heart moves.

   (c) is in the posterior area of the thoracic cavity.

   (d) Both answers (a) and (c).

   (e) Both answers (b) and (c).

246. The pericardium

   (a) contains the heart, large blood vessels, and parts of the trachea and esophagus.

   (b) surrounds the heart and contains a small amount of fluid that prevents friction as the heart moves.

   (c) is in the posterior area of the thoracic cavity.

   (d) Both answers (a) and (c).

   (e) Both answers (b) and (c).

247. The largest gland in the body is the

   (a) brain.

   (b) gallbladder.

   (c) pancreas.

   (d) lungs.

   (e) liver.

248. Insulin and digestive juices are produced in the

    (a) brain.

    (b) gallbladder.

    (c) pancreas.

    (d) lungs.

    (e) liver.

249. Priapism is caused by

    (a) peritonitis that produces abnormal muscle activity.

    (b) head injury that produces small, rarely detectable, seizures.

    (c) spinal cord injury.

    (d) All of the above.

    (e) None of the above.

250. Projectile vomiting frequently accompanies serious head injury and is defined as

    (a) emesis containing sharp, dangerous material.

    (b) forceful ejection of vomitus, frequently without warning.

    (c) nausea, vomiting, and diarrhea.

    (d) All of the above.

    (e) None of the above.

The answer key for Test Section Four is on page 230.

TEST SECTION ONE ANSWER SHEET

1.	(a)	(b)	(c)	(d)	(e)	43.	(a)	(b)	(c)	(d)	(e)
2.	(a)	(b)	(c)	(d)	(e)	44.	(a)	(b)	(c)	(d)	(e)
3.	(a)	(b)	(c)	(d)	(e)	45.	(a)	(b)	(c)	(d)	(e)
4.	(a)	(b)	(c)	(d)	(e)	46.	(a)	(b)	(c)	(d)	(e)
5.	(a)	(b)	(c)	(d)	(e)	47.	(a)	(b)	(c)	(d)	(e)
6.	(a)	(b)	(c)	(d)	(e)	48.	(a)	(b)	(c)	(d)	(e)
7.	(a)	(b)	(c)	(d)	(e)	49.	(a)	(b)	(c)	(d)	(e)
8.	(a)	(b)	(c)	(d)	(e)	50.	(a)	(b)	(c)	(d)	(e)
9.	(a)	(b)	(c)	(d)	(e)	51.	(a)	(b)	(c)	(d)	(e)
10.	(a)	(b)	(c)	(d)	(e)	52.	(a)	(b)	(c)	(d)	(e)
11.	(a)	(b)	(c)	(d)	(e)	53.	(a)	(b)	(c)	(d)	(e)
12.	(a)	(b)	(c)	(d)	(e)	54.	(a)	(b)	(c)	(d)	(e)
13.	(a)	(b)	(c)	(d)	(e)	55.	(a)	(b)	(c)	(d)	(e)
14.	(a)	(b)	(c)	(d)	(e)	56.	(a)	(b)	(c)	(d)	(e)
15.	(a)	(b)	(c)	(d)	(e)	57.	(a)	(b)	(c)	(d)	(e)
16.	(a)	(b)	(c)	(d)	(e)	58.	(a)	(b)	(c)	(d)	(e)
17.	(a)	(b)	(c)	(d)	(e)	59.	(a)	(b)	(c)	(d)	(e)
18.	(a)	(b)	(c)	(d)	(e)	60.	(a)	(b)	(c)	(d)	(e)
19.	(a)	(b)	(c)	(d)	(e)	61.	(a)	(b)	(c)	(d)	(e)
20.	(a)	(b)	(c)	(d)	(e)	62.	(a)	(b)	(c)	(d)	(e)
21.	(a)	(b)	(c)	(d)	(e)	63.	(a)	(b)	(c)	(d)	(e)
22.	(a)	(b)	(c)	(d)	(e)	64.	(a)	(b)	(c)	(d)	(e)
23.	(a)	(b)	(c)	(d)	(e)	65.	(a)	(b)	(c)	(d)	(e)
24.	(a)	(b)	(c)	(d)	(e)	66.	(a)	(b)	(c)	(d)	(e)
25.	(a)	(b)	(c)	(d)	(e)	67.	(a)	(b)	(c)	(d)	(e)
26.	(a)	(b)	(c)	(d)	(e)	68.	(a)	(b)	(c)	(d)	(e)
27.	(a)	(b)	(c)	(d)	(e)	69.	(a)	(b)	(c)	(d)	(e)
28.	(a)	(b)	(c)	(d)	(e)	70.	(a)	(b)	(c)	(d)	(e)
29.	(a)	(b)	(c)	(d)	(e)	71.	(a)	(b)	(c)	(d)	(e)
30.	(a)	(b)	(c)	(d)	(e)	72.	(a)	(b)	(c)	(d)	(e)
31.	(a)	(b)	(c)	(d)	(e)	73.	(a)	(b)	(c)	(d)	(e)
32.	(a)	(b)	(c)	(d)	(e)	74.	(a)	(b)	(c)	(d)	(e)
33.	(a)	(b)	(c)	(d)	(e)	75.	(a)	(b)	(c)	(d)	(e)
34.	(a)	(b)	(c)	(d)	(e)	76.	(a)	(b)	(c)	(d)	(e)
35.	(a)	(b)	(c)	(d)	(e)	77.	(a)	(b)	(c)	(d)	(e)
36.	(a)	(b)	(c)	(d)	(e)	78.	(a)	(b)	(c)	(d)	(e)
37.	(a)	(b)	(c)	(d)	(e)	79.	(a)	(b)	(c)	(d)	(e)
38.	(a)	(b)	(c)	(d)	(e)	80.	(a)	(b)	(c)	(d)	(e)
39.	(a)	(b)	(c)	(d)	(e)	81.	(a)	(b)	(c)	(d)	(e)
40.	(a)	(b)	(c)	(d)	(e)	82.	(a)	(b)	(c)	(d)	(e)
41.	(a)	(b)	(c)	(d)	(e)	83.	(a)	(b)	(c)	(d)	(e)
42.	(a)	(b)	(c)	(d)	(e)	84.	(a)	(b)	(c)	(d)	(e)

85.	(a)	(b)	(c)	(d)	(e)
86.	(a)	(b)	(c)	(d)	(e)
87.	(a)	(b)	(c)	(d)	(e)
88.	(a)	(b)	(c)	(d)	(e)
89.	(a)	(b)	(c)	(d)	(e)
90.	(a)	(b)	(c)	(d)	(e)
91.	(a)	(b)	(c)	(d)	(e)
92.	(a)	(b)	(c)	(d)	(e)
93.	(a)	(b)	(c)	(d)	(e)
94.	(a)	(b)	(c)	(d)	(e)
95.	(a)	(b)	(c)	(d)	(e)
96.	(a)	(b)	(c)	(d)	(e)
97.	(a)	(b)	(c)	(d)	(e)
98.	(a)	(b)	(c)	(d)	(e)
99.	(a)	(b)	(c)	(d)	(e)
100.	(a)	(b)	(c)	(d)	(e)
101.	(a)	(b)	(c)	(d)	(e)
102.	(a)	(b)	(c)	(d)	(e)
103.	(a)	(b)	(c)	(d)	(e)
104.	(a)	(b)	(c)	(d)	(e)
105.	(a)	(b)	(c)	(d)	(e)
106.	(a)	(b)	(c)	(d)	(e)
107.	(a)	(b)	(c)	(d)	(e)
108.	(a)	(b)	(c)	(d)	(e)
109.	(a)	(b)	(c)	(d)	(e)
110.	(a)	(b)	(c)	(d)	(e)
111.	(a)	(b)	(c)	(d)	(e)
112.	(a)	(b)	(c)	(d)	(e)
113.	(a)	(b)	(c)	(d)	(e)
114.	(a)	(b)	(c)	(d)	(e)
115.	(a)	(b)	(c)	(d)	(e)
116.	(a)	(b)	(c)	(d)	(e)
117.	(a)	(b)	(c)	(d)	(e)
118.	(a)	(b)	(c)	(d)	(e)
119.	(a)	(b)	(c)	(d)	(e)
120.	(a)	(b)	(c)	(d)	(e)
121.	(a)	(b)	(c)	(d)	(e)
122.	(a)	(b)	(c)	(d)	(e)
123.	(a)	(b)	(c)	(d)	(e)
124.	(a)	(b)	(c)	(d)	(e)
125.	(a)	(b)	(c)	(d)	(e)
126.	(a)	(b)	(c)	(d)	(e)
127.	(a)	(b)	(c)	(d)	(e)
128.	(a)	(b)	(c)	(d)	(e)
129.	(a)	(b)	(c)	(d)	(e)
130.	(a)	(b)	(c)	(d)	(e)
131.	(a)	(b)	(c)	(d)	(e)

132.	(a)	(b)	(c)	(d)	(e)
133.	(a)	(b)	(c)	(d)	(e)
134.	(a)	(b)	(c)	(d)	(e)
135.	(a)	(b)	(c)	(d)	(e)
136.	(a)	(b)	(c)	(d)	(e)
137.	(a)	(b)	(c)	(d)	(e)
138.	(a)	(b)	(c)	(d)	(e)
139.	(a)	(b)	(c)	(d)	(e)

TEST SECTION TWO ANSWER SHEET

1.	(a)	(b)	(c)	(d)	(e)	43.	(a)	(b)	(c)	(d)	(e)
2.	(a)	(b)	(c)	(d)	(e)	44.	(a)	(b)	(c)	(d)	(e)
3.	(a)	(b)	(c)	(d)	(e)	45.	(a)	(b)	(c)	(d)	(e)
4.	(a)	(b)	(c)	(d)	(e)	46.	(a)	(b)	(c)	(d)	(e)
5.	(a)	(b)	(c)	(d)	(e)	47.	(a)	(b)	(c)	(d)	(e)
6.	(a)	(b)	(c)	(d)	(e)	48.	(a)	(b)	(c)	(d)	(e)
7.	(a)	(b)	(c)	(d)	(e)	49.	(a)	(b)	(c)	(d)	(e)
8.	(a)	(b)	(c)	(d)	(e)	50.	(a)	(b)	(c)	(d)	(e)
9.	(a)	(b)	(c)	(d)	(e)	51.	(a)	(b)	(c)	(d)	(e)
10.	(a)	(b)	(c)	(d)	(e)	52.	(a)	(b)	(c)	(d)	(e)
11.	(a)	(b)	(c)	(d)	(e)	53.	(a)	(b)	(c)	(d)	(e)
12.	(a)	(b)	(c)	(d)	(e)	54.	(a)	(b)	(c)	(d)	(e)
13.	(a)	(b)	(c)	(d)	(e)	55.	(a)	(b)	(c)	(d)	(e)
14.	(a)	(b)	(c)	(d)	(e)	56.	(a)	(b)	(c)	(d)	(e)
15.	(a)	(b)	(c)	(d)	(e)	57.	(a)	(b)	(c)	(d)	(e)
16.	(a)	(b)	(c)	(d)	(e)	58.	(a)	(b)	(c)	(d)	(e)
17.	(a)	(b)	(c)	(d)	(e)	59.	(a)	(b)	(c)	(d)	(e)
18.	(a)	(b)	(c)	(d)	(e)	60.	(a)	(b)	(c)	(d)	(e)
19.	(a)	(b)	(c)	(d)	(e)	61.	(a)	(b)	(c)	(d)	(e)
20.	(a)	(b)	(c)	(d)	(e)	62.	(a)	(b)	(c)	(d)	(e)
21.	(a)	(b)	(c)	(d)	(e)	63.	(a)	(b)	(c)	(d)	(e)
22.	(a)	(b)	(c)	(d)	(e)	64.	(a)	(b)	(c)	(d)	(e)
23.	(a)	(b)	(c)	(d)	(e)	65.	(a)	(b)	(c)	(d)	(e)
24.	(a)	(b)	(c)	(d)	(e)	66.	(a)	(b)	(c)	(d)	(e)
25.	(a)	(b)	(c)	(d)	(e)	67.	(a)	(b)	(c)	(d)	(e)
26.	(a)	(b)	(c)	(d)	(e)	68.	(a)	(b)	(c)	(d)	(e)
27.	(a)	(b)	(c)	(d)	(e)	69.	(a)	(b)	(c)	(d)	(e)
28.	(a)	(b)	(c)	(d)	(e)	70.	(a)	(b)	(c)	(d)	(e)
29.	(a)	(b)	(c)	(d)	(e)	71.	(a)	(b)	(c)	(d)	(e)
30.	(a)	(b)	(c)	(d)	(e)	72.	(a)	(b)	(c)	(d)	(e)
31.	(a)	(b)	(c)	(d)	(e)	73.	(a)	(b)	(c)	(d)	(e)
32.	(a)	(b)	(c)	(d)	(e)	74.	(a)	(b)	(c)	(d)	(e)
33.	(a)	(b)	(c)	(d)	(e)	75.	(a)	(b)	(c)	(d)	(e)
34.	(a)	(b)	(c)	(d)	(e)	76.	(a)	(b)	(c)	(d)	(e)
35.	(a)	(b)	(c)	(d)	(e)	77.	(a)	(b)	(c)	(d)	(e)
36.	(a)	(b)	(c)	(d)	(e)	78.	(a)	(b)	(c)	(d)	(e)
37.	(a)	(b)	(c)	(d)	(e)	79.	(a)	(b)	(c)	(d)	(e)
38.	(a)	(b)	(c)	(d)	(e)	80.	(a)	(b)	(c)	(d)	(e)
39.	(a)	(b)	(c)	(d)	(e)	81.	(a)	(b)	(c)	(d)	(e)
40.	(a)	(b)	(c)	(d)	(e)	82.	(a)	(b)	(c)	(d)	(e)
41.	(a)	(b)	(c)	(d)	(e)	83.	(a)	(b)	(c)	(d)	(e)
42.	(a)	(b)	(c)	(d)	(e)	84.	(a)	(b)	(c)	(d)	(e)

85.	(a)	(b)	(c)	(d)	(e)	132.	(a)	(b)	(c)	(d)	(e)
86.	(a)	(b)	(c)	(d)	(e)	133.	(a)	(b)	(c)	(d)	(e)
87.	(a)	(b)	(c)	(d)	(e)	134.	(a)	(b)	(c)	(d)	(e)
88.	(a)	(b)	(c)	(d)	(e)	135.	(a)	(b)	(c)	(d)	(e)
89.	(a)	(b)	(c)	(d)	(e)	136.	(a)	(b)	(c)	(d)	(e)
90.	(a)	(b)	(c)	(d)	(e)	137.	(a)	(b)	(c)	(d)	(e)
91.	(a)	(b)	(c)	(d)	(e)	138.	(a)	(b)	(c)	(d)	(e)
92.	(a)	(b)	(c)	(d)	(e)	139.	(a)	(b)	(c)	(d)	(e)
93.	(a)	(b)	(c)	(d)	(e)	140.	(a)	(b)	(c)	(d)	(e)
94.	(a)	(b)	(c)	(d)	(e)	141.	(a)	(b)	(c)	(d)	(e)
95.	(a)	(b)	(c)	(d)	(e)	142.	(a)	(b)	(c)	(d)	(e)
96.	(a)	(b)	(c)	(d)	(e)	143.	(a)	(b)	(c)	(d)	(e)
97.	(a)	(b)	(c)	(d)	(e)	144.	(a)	(b)	(c)	(d)	(e)
98.	(a)	(b)	(c)	(d)	(e)	145.	(a)	(b)	(c)	(d)	(e)
99.	(a)	(b)	(c)	(d)	(e)	146.	(a)	(b)	(c)	(d)	(e)
100.	(a)	(b)	(c)	(d)	(e)	147.	(a)	(b)	(c)	(d)	(e)
101.	(a)	(b)	(c)	(d)	(e)	148.	(a)	(b)	(c)	(d)	(e)
102.	(a)	(b)	(c)	(d)	(e)	149.	(a)	(b)	(c)	(d)	(e)
103.	(a)	(b)	(c)	(d)	(e)	150.	(a)	(b)	(c)	(d)	(e)
104.	(a)	(b)	(c)	(d)	(e)	151.	(a)	(b)	(c)	(d)	(e)
105.	(a)	(b)	(c)	(d)	(e)	152.	(a)	(b)	(c)	(d)	(e)
106.	(a)	(b)	(c)	(d)	(e)	153.	(a)	(b)	(c)	(d)	(e)
107.	(a)	(b)	(c)	(d)	(e)	154.	(a)	(b)	(c)	(d)	(e)
108.	(a)	(b)	(c)	(d)	(e)	155.	(a)	(b)	(c)	(d)	(e)
109.	(a)	(b)	(c)	(d)	(e)	156.	(a)	(b)	(c)	(d)	(e)
110.	(a)	(b)	(c)	(d)	(e)	157.	(a)	(b)	(c)	(d)	(e)
111.	(a)	(b)	(c)	(d)	(e)	158.	(a)	(b)	(c)	(d)	(e)
112.	(a)	(b)	(c)	(d)	(e)	159.	(a)	(b)	(c)	(d)	(e)
113.	(a)	(b)	(c)	(d)	(e)	160.	(a)	(b)	(c)	(d)	(e)
114.	(a)	(b)	(c)	(d)	(e)	161.	(a)	(b)	(c)	(d)	(e)
115.	(a)	(b)	(c)	(d)	(e)	162.	(a)	(b)	(c)	(d)	(e)
116.	(a)	(b)	(c)	(d)	(e)	163.	(a)	(b)	(c)	(d)	(e)
117.	(a)	(b)	(c)	(d)	(e)	164.	(a)	(b)	(c)	(d)	(e)
118.	(a)	(b)	(c)	(d)	(e)	165.	(a)	(b)	(c)	(d)	(e)
119.	(a)	(b)	(c)	(d)	(e)	166.	(a)	(b)	(c)	(d)	(e)
120.	(a)	(b)	(c)	(d)	(e)	167.	(a)	(b)	(c)	(d)	(e)
121.	(a)	(b)	(c)	(d)	(e)	168.	(a)	(b)	(c)	(d)	(e)
122.	(a)	(b)	(c)	(d)	(e)	169.	(a)	(b)	(c)	(d)	(e)
123.	(a)	(b)	(c)	(d)	(e)	170.	(a)	(b)	(c)	(d)	(e)
124.	(a)	(b)	(c)	(d)	(e)	171.	(a)	(b)	(c)	(d)	(e)
125.	(a)	(b)	(c)	(d)	(e)	172.	(a)	(b)	(c)	(d)	(e)
126.	(a)	(b)	(c)	(d)	(e)	173.	(a)	(b)	(c)	(d)	(e)
127.	(a)	(b)	(c)	(d)	(e)	174.	(a)	(b)	(c)	(d)	(e)
128.	(a)	(b)	(c)	(d)	(e)	175.	(a)	(b)	(c)	(d)	(e)
129.	(a)	(b)	(c)	(d)	(e)	176.	(a)	(b)	(c)	(d)	(e)
130.	(a)	(b)	(c)	(d)	(e)	177.	(a)	(b)	(c)	(d)	(e)
131.	(a)	(b)	(c)	(d)	(e)	178.	(a)	(b)	(c)	(d)	(e)

179.	(a)	(b)	(c)	(d)	(e)	226.	(a)	(b)	(c)	(d)	(e)
180.	(a)	(b)	(c)	(d)	(e)	227.	(a)	(b)	(c)	(d)	(e)
181.	(a)	(b)	(c)	(d)	(e)	228.	(a)	(b)	(c)	(d)	(e)
182.	(a)	(b)	(c)	(d)	(e)	229.	(a)	(b)	(c)	(d)	(e)
183.	(a)	(b)	(c)	(d)	(e)	230.	(a)	(b)	(c)	(d)	(e)
184.	(a)	(b)	(c)	(d)	(e)	231.	(a)	(b)	(c)	(d)	(e)
185.	(a)	(b)	(c)	(d)	(e)	232.	(a)	(b)	(c)	(d)	(e)
186.	(a)	(b)	(c)	(d)	(e)	233.	(a)	(b)	(c)	(d)	(e)
187.	(a)	(b)	(c)	(d)	(e)	234.	(a)	(b)	(c)	(d)	(e)
188.	(a)	(b)	(c)	(d)	(e)	235.	(a)	(b)	(c)	(d)	(e)
189.	(a)	(b)	(c)	(d)	(e)	236.	(a)	(b)	(c)	(d)	(e)
190.	(a)	(b)	(c)	(d)	(e)	237.	(a)	(b)	(c)	(d)	(e)
191.	(a)	(b)	(c)	(d)	(e)	238.	(a)	(b)	(c)	(d)	(e)
192.	(a)	(b)	(c)	(d)	(e)	239.	(a)	(b)	(c)	(d)	(e)
193.	(a)	(b)	(c)	(d)	(e)	240.	(a)	(b)	(c)	(d)	(e)
194.	(a)	(b)	(c)	(d)	(e)	241.	(a)	(b)	(c)	(d)	(e)
195.	(a)	(b)	(c)	(d)	(e)	242.	(a)	(b)	(c)	(d)	(e)
196.	(a)	(b)	(c)	(d)	(e)	243.	(a)	(b)	(c)	(d)	(e)
197.	(a)	(b)	(c)	(d)	(e)	244.	(a)	(b)	(c)	(d)	(e)
198.	(a)	(b)	(c)	(d)	(e)	245.	(a)	(b)	(c)	(d)	(e)
199.	(a)	(b)	(c)	(d)	(e)	246.	(a)	(b)	(c)	(d)	(e)
200.	(a)	(b)	(c)	(d)	(e)	247.	(a)	(b)	(c)	(d)	(e)
201.	(a)	(b)	(c)	(d)	(e)	248.	(a)	(b)	(c)	(d)	(e)
202.	(a)	(b)	(c)	(d)	(e)	249.	(a)	(b)	(c)	(d)	(e)
203.	(a)	(b)	(c)	(d)	(e)	250.	(a)	(b)	(c)	(d)	(e)
204.	(a)	(b)	(c)	(d)	(e)	251.	(a)	(b)	(c)	(d)	(e)
205.	(a)	(b)	(c)	(d)	(e)	252.	(a)	(b)	(c)	(d)	(e)
206.	(a)	(b)	(c)	(d)	(e)	253.	(a)	(b)	(c)	(d)	(e)
207.	(a)	(b)	(c)	(d)	(e)	254.	(a)	(b)	(c)	(d)	(e)
208.	(a)	(b)	(c)	(d)	(e)	255.	(a)	(b)	(c)	(d)	(e)
209.	(a)	(b)	(c)	(d)	(e)	256.	(a)	(b)	(c)	(d)	(e)
210.	(a)	(b)	(c)	(d)	(e)	257.	(a)	(b)	(c)	(d)	(e)
211.	(a)	(b)	(c)	(d)	(e)	258.	(a)	(b)	(c)	(d)	(e)
212.	(a)	(b)	(c)	(d)	(e)	259.	(a)	(b)	(c)	(d)	(e)
213.	(a)	(b)	(c)	(d)	(e)	260.	(a)	(b)	(c)	(d)	(e)
214.	(a)	(b)	(c)	(d)	(e)	261.	(a)	(b)	(c)	(d)	(e)
215.	(a)	(b)	(c)	(d)	(e)	262.	(a)	(b)	(c)	(d)	(e)
216.	(a)	(b)	(c)	(d)	(e)	263.	(a)	(b)	(c)	(d)	(e)
217.	(a)	(b)	(c)	(d)	(e)	264.	(a)	(b)	(c)	(d)	(e)
218.	(a)	(b)	(c)	(d)	(e)	265.	(a)	(b)	(c)	(d)	(e)
219.	(a)	(b)	(c)	(d)	(e)	266.	(a)	(b)	(c)	(d)	(e)
220.	(a)	(b)	(c)	(d)	(e)	267.	(a)	(b)	(c)	(d)	(e)
221.	(a)	(b)	(c)	(d)	(e)	268.	(a)	(b)	(c)	(d)	(e)
222.	(a)	(b)	(c)	(d)	(e)	269.	(a)	(b)	(c)	(d)	(e)
223.	(a)	(b)	(c)	(d)	(e)	270.	(a)	(b)	(c)	(d)	(e)
224.	(a)	(b)	(c)	(d)	(e)	271.	(a)	(b)	(c)	(d)	(e)
225.	(a)	(b)	(c)	(d)	(e)	272.	(a)	(b)	(c)	(d)	(e)

TEST SECTION THREE ANSWER SHEET

1.	(a)	(b)	(c)	(d)	(e)	43.	(a)	(b)	(c)	(d)	(e)
2.	(a)	(b)	(c)	(d)	(e)	44.	(a)	(b)	(c)	(d)	(e)
3.	(a)	(b)	(c)	(d)	(e)	45.	(a)	(b)	(c)	(d)	(e)
4.	(a)	(b)	(c)	(d)	(e)	46.	(a)	(b)	(c)	(d)	(e)
5.	(a)	(b)	(c)	(d)	(e)	47.	(a)	(b)	(c)	(d)	(e)
6.	(a)	(b)	(c)	(d)	(e)	48.	(a)	(b)	(c)	(d)	(e)
7.	(a)	(b)	(c)	(d)	(e)	49.	(a)	(b)	(c)	(d)	(e)
8.	(a)	(b)	(c)	(d)	(e)	50.	(a)	(b)	(c)	(d)	(e)
9.	(a)	(b)	(c)	(d)	(e)	51.	(a)	(b)	(c)	(d)	(e)
10.	(a)	(b)	(c)	(d)	(e)	52.	(a)	(b)	(c)	(d)	(e)
11.	(a)	(b)	(c)	(d)	(e)	53.	(a)	(b)	(c)	(d)	(e)
12.	(a)	(b)	(c)	(d)	(e)	54.	(a)	(b)	(c)	(d)	(e)
13.	(a)	(b)	(c)	(d)	(e)	55.	(a)	(b)	(c)	(d)	(e)
14.	(a)	(b)	(c)	(d)	(e)	56.	(a)	(b)	(c)	(d)	(e)
15.	(a)	(b)	(c)	(d)	(e)	57.	(a)	(b)	(c)	(d)	(e)
16.	(a)	(b)	(c)	(d)	(e)	58.	(a)	(b)	(c)	(d)	(e)
17.	(a)	(b)	(c)	(d)	(e)	59.	(a)	(b)	(c)	(d)	(e)
18.	(a)	(b)	(c)	(d)	(e)	60.	(a)	(b)	(c)	(d)	(e)
19.	(a)	(b)	(c)	(d)	(e)	61.	(a)	(b)	(c)	(d)	(e)
20.	(a)	(b)	(c)	(d)	(e)	62.	(a)	(b)	(c)	(d)	(e)
21.	(a)	(b)	(c)	(d)	(e)	63.	(a)	(b)	(c)	(d)	(e)
22.	(a)	(b)	(c)	(d)	(e)	64.	(a)	(b)	(c)	(d)	(e)
23.	(a)	(b)	(c)	(d)	(e)	65.	(a)	(b)	(c)	(d)	(e)
24.	(a)	(b)	(c)	(d)	(e)	66.	(a)	(b)	(c)	(d)	(e)
25.	(a)	(b)	(c)	(d)	(e)	67.	(a)	(b)	(c)	(d)	(e)
26.	(a)	(b)	(c)	(d)	(e)	68.	(a)	(b)	(c)	(d)	(e)
27.	(a)	(b)	(c)	(d)	(e)	69.	(a)	(b)	(c)	(d)	(e)
28.	(a)	(b)	(c)	(d)	(e)	70.	(a)	(b)	(c)	(d)	(e)
29.	(a)	(b)	(c)	(d)	(e)	71.	(a)	(b)	(c)	(d)	(e)
30.	(a)	(b)	(c)	(d)	(e)	72.	(a)	(b)	(c)	(d)	(e)
31.	(a)	(b)	(c)	(d)	(e)	73.	(a)	(b)	(c)	(d)	(e)
32.	(a)	(b)	(c)	(d)	(e)	74.	(a)	(b)	(c)	(d)	(e)
33.	(a)	(b)	(c)	(d)	(e)	75.	(a)	(b)	(c)	(d)	(e)
34.	(a)	(b)	(c)	(d)	(e)	76.	(a)	(b)	(c)	(d)	(e)
35.	(a)	(b)	(c)	(d)	(e)	77.	(a)	(b)	(c)	(d)	(e)
36.	(a)	(b)	(c)	(d)	(e)	78.	(a)	(b)	(c)	(d)	(e)
37.	(a)	(b)	(c)	(d)	(e)	79.	(a)	(b)	(c)	(d)	(e)
38.	(a)	(b)	(c)	(d)	(e)	80.	(a)	(b)	(c)	(d)	(e)
39.	(a)	(b)	(c)	(d)	(e)	81.	(a)	(b)	(c)	(d)	(e)
40.	(a)	(b)	(c)	(d)	(e)	82.	(a)	(b)	(c)	(d)	(e)
41.	(a)	(b)	(c)	(d)	(e)	83.	(a)	(b)	(c)	(d)	(e)
42.	(a)	(b)	(c)	(d)	(e)	84.	(a)	(b)	(c)	(d)	(e)

206

TEST SECTION THREE ANSWER SHEET

85.	(a)	(b)	(c)	(d)	(e)	132.	(a)	(b)	(c)	(d)	(e)
86.	(a)	(b)	(c)	(d)	(e)	133.	(a)	(b)	(c)	(d)	(e)
87.	(a)	(b)	(c)	(d)	(e)	134.	(a)	(b)	(c)	(d)	(e)
88.	(a)	(b)	(c)	(d)	(e)	135.	(a)	(b)	(c)	(d)	(e)
89.	(a)	(b)	(c)	(d)	(e)	136.	(a)	(b)	(c)	(d)	(e)
90.	(a)	(b)	(c)	(d)	(e)	137.	(a)	(b)	(c)	(d)	(e)
91.	(a)	(b)	(c)	(d)	(e)	138.	(a)	(b)	(c)	(d)	(e)
92.	(a)	(b)	(c)	(d)	(e)	139.	(a)	(b)	(c)	(d)	(e)
93.	(a)	(b)	(c)	(d)	(e)	140.	(a)	(b)	(c)	(d)	(e)
94.	(a)	(b)	(c)	(d)	(e)	141.	(a)	(b)	(c)	(d)	(e)
95.	(a)	(b)	(c)	(d)	(e)	142.	(a)	(b)	(c)	(d)	(e)
96.	(a)	(b)	(c)	(d)	(e)	143.	(a)	(b)	(c)	(d)	(e)
97.	(a)	(b)	(c)	(d)	(e)	144.	(a)	(b)	(c)	(d)	(e)
98.	(a)	(b)	(c)	(d)	(e)	145.	(a)	(b)	(c)	(d)	(e)
99.	(a)	(b)	(c)	(d)	(e)	146.	(a)	(b)	(c)	(d)	(e)
100.	(a)	(b)	(c)	(d)	(e)	147.	(a)	(b)	(c)	(d)	(e)
101.	(a)	(b)	(c)	(d)	(e)	148.	(a)	(b)	(c)	(d)	(e)
102.	(a)	(b)	(c)	(d)	(e)	149.	(a)	(b)	(c)	(d)	(e)
103.	(a)	(b)	(c)	(d)	(e)	150.	(a)	(b)	(c)	(d)	(e)
104.	(a)	(b)	(c)	(d)	(e)	151.	(a)	(b)	(c)	(d)	(e)
105.	(a)	(b)	(c)	(d)	(e)	152.	(a)	(b)	(c)	(d)	(e)
106.	(a)	(b)	(c)	(d)	(e)	153.	(a)	(b)	(c)	(d)	(e)
107.	(a)	(b)	(c)	(d)	(e)	154.	(a)	(b)	(c)	(d)	(e)
108.	(a)	(b)	(c)	(d)	(e)	155.	(a)	(b)	(c)	(d)	(e)
109.	(a)	(b)	(c)	(d)	(e)	156.	(a)	(b)	(c)	(d)	(e)
110.	(a)	(b)	(c)	(d)	(e)	157.	(a)	(b)	(c)	(d)	(e)
111.	(a)	(b)	(c)	(d)	(e)	158.	(a)	(b)	(c)	(d)	(e)
112.	(a)	(b)	(c)	(d)	(e)	159.	(a)	(b)	(c)	(d)	(e)
113.	(a)	(b)	(c)	(d)	(e)	160.	(a)	(b)	(c)	(d)	(e)
114.	(a)	(b)	(c)	(d)	(e)	161.	(a)	(b)	(c)	(d)	(e)
115.	(a)	(b)	(c)	(d)	(e)	162.	(a)	(b)	(c)	(d)	(e)
116.	(a)	(b)	(c)	(d)	(e)	163.	(a)	(b)	(c)	(d)	(e)
117.	(a)	(b)	(c)	(d)	(e)	164.	(a)	(b)	(c)	(d)	(e)
118.	(a)	(b)	(c)	(d)	(e)	165.	(a)	(b)	(c)	(d)	(e)
119.	(a)	(b)	(c)	(d)	(e)	166.	(a)	(b)	(c)	(d)	(e)
120.	(a)	(b)	(c)	(d)	(e)	167.	(a)	(b)	(c)	(d)	(e)
121.	(a)	(b)	(c)	(d)	(e)	168.	(a)	(b)	(c)	(d)	(e)
122.	(a)	(b)	(c)	(d)	(e)	169.	(a)	(b)	(c)	(d)	(e)
123.	(a)	(b)	(c)	(d)	(e)	170.	(a)	(b)	(c)	(d)	(e)
124.	(a)	(b)	(c)	(d)	(e)	171.	(a)	(b)	(c)	(d)	(e)
125.	(a)	(b)	(c)	(d)	(e)	172.	(a)	(b)	(c)	(d)	(e)
126.	(a)	(b)	(c)	(d)	(e)	173.	(a)	(b)	(c)	(d)	(e)
127.	(a)	(b)	(c)	(d)	(e)	174.	(a)	(b)	(c)	(d)	(e)
128.	(a)	(b)	(c)	(d)	(e)	175.	(a)	(b)	(c)	(d)	(e)
129.	(a)	(b)	(c)	(d)	(e)	176.	(a)	(b)	(c)	(d)	(e)
130.	(a)	(b)	(c)	(d)	(e)	177.	(a)	(b)	(c)	(d)	(e)
131.	(a)	(b)	(c)	(d)	(e)	178.	(a)	(b)	(c)	(d)	(e)

179.	(a)	(b)	(c)	(d)	(e)	226.	(a)	(b)	(c)	(d)	(e)
180.	(a)	(b)	(c)	(d)	(e)	227.	(a)	(b)	(c)	(d)	(e)
181.	(a)	(b)	(c)	(d)	(e)	228.	(a)	(b)	(c)	(d)	(e)
182.	(a)	(b)	(c)	(d)	(e)	229.	(a)	(b)	(c)	(d)	(e)
183.	(a)	(b)	(c)	(d)	(e)	230.	(a)	(b)	(c)	(d)	(e)
184.	(a)	(b)	(c)	(d)	(e)	231.	(a)	(b)	(c)	(d)	(e)
185.	(a)	(b)	(c)	(d)	(e)	232.	(a)	(b)	(c)	(d)	(e)
186.	(a)	(b)	(c)	(d)	(e)	233.	(a)	(b)	(c)	(d)	(e)
187.	(a)	(b)	(c)	(d)	(e)	234.	(a)	(b)	(c)	(d)	(e)
188.	(a)	(b)	(c)	(d)	(e)	235.	(a)	(b)	(c)	(d)	(e)
189.	(a)	(b)	(c)	(d)	(e)	236.	(a)	(b)	(c)	(d)	(e)
190.	(a)	(b)	(c)	(d)	(e)	237.	(a)	(b)	(c)	(d)	(e)
191.	(a)	(b)	(c)	(d)	(e)	238.	(a)	(b)	(c)	(d)	(e)
192.	(a)	(b)	(c)	(d)	(e)	239.	(a)	(b)	(c)	(d)	(e)
193.	(a)	(b)	(c)	(d)	(e)	240.	(a)	(b)	(c)	(d)	(e)
194.	(a)	(b)	(c)	(d)	(e)	241.	(a)	(b)	(c)	(d)	(e)
195.	(a)	(b)	(c)	(d)	(e)	242.	(a)	(b)	(c)	(d)	(e)
196.	(a)	(b)	(c)	(d)	(e)	243.	(a)	(b)	(c)	(d)	(e)
197.	(a)	(b)	(c)	(d)	(e)	244.	(a)	(b)	(c)	(d)	(e)
198.	(a)	(b)	(c)	(d)	(e)	245.	(a)	(b)	(c)	(d)	(e)
199.	(a)	(b)	(c)	(d)	(e)	246.	(a)	(b)	(c)	(d)	(e)
200.	(a)	(b)	(c)	(d)	(e)	247.	(a)	(b)	(c)	(d)	(e)
201.	(a)	(b)	(c)	(d)	(e)	248.	(a)	(b)	(c)	(d)	(e)
202.	(a)	(b)	(c)	(d)	(e)	249.	(a)	(b)	(c)	(d)	(e)
203.	(a)	(b)	(c)	(d)	(e)	250.	(a)	(b)	(c)	(d)	(e)
204.	(a)	(b)	(c)	(d)	(e)	251.	(a)	(b)	(c)	(d)	(e)
205.	(a)	(b)	(c)	(d)	(e)	252.	(a)	(b)	(c)	(d)	(e)
206.	(a)	(b)	(c)	(d)	(e)	253.	(a)	(b)	(c)	(d)	(e)
207.	(a)	(b)	(c)	(d)	(e)	254.	(a)	(b)	(c)	(d)	(e)
208.	(a)	(b)	(c)	(d)	(e)	255.	(a)	(b)	(c)	(d)	(e)
209.	(a)	(b)	(c)	(d)	(e)	256.	(a)	(b)	(c)	(d)	(e)
210.	(a)	(b)	(c)	(d)	(e)	257.	(a)	(b)	(c)	(d)	(e)
211.	(a)	(b)	(c)	(d)	(e)						
212.	(a)	(b)	(c)	(d)	(e)						
213.	(a)	(b)	(c)	(d)	(e)						
214.	(a)	(b)	(c)	(d)	(e)						
215.	(a)	(b)	(c)	(d)	(e)						
216.	(a)	(b)	(c)	(d)	(e)						
217.	(a)	(b)	(c)	(d)	(e)						
218.	(a)	(b)	(c)	(d)	(e)						
219.	(a)	(b)	(c)	(d)	(e)						
220.	(a)	(b)	(c)	(d)	(e)						
221.	(a)	(b)	(c)	(d)	(e)						
222.	(a)	(b)	(c)	(d)	(e)						
223.	(a)	(b)	(c)	(d)	(e)						
224.	(a)	(b)	(c)	(d)	(e)						
225.	(a)	(b)	(c)	(d)	(e)						

TEST SECTION FOUR ANSWER SHEET

1.	(a)	(b)	(c)	(d)	(e)	43.	(a)	(b)	(c)	(d)	(e)
2.	(a)	(b)	(c)	(d)	(e)	44.	(a)	(b)	(c)	(d)	(e)
3.	(a)	(b)	(c)	(d)	(e)	45.	(a)	(b)	(c)	(d)	(e)
4.	(a)	(b)	(c)	(d)	(e)	46.	(a)	(b)	(c)	(d)	(e)
5.	(a)	(b)	(c)	(d)	(e)	47.	(a)	(b)	(c)	(d)	(e)
6.	(a)	(b)	(c)	(d)	(e)	48.	(a)	(b)	(c)	(d)	(e)
7.	(a)	(b)	(c)	(d)	(e)	49.	(a)	(b)	(c)	(d)	(e)
8.	(a)	(b)	(c)	(d)	(e)	50.	(a)	(b)	(c)	(d)	(e)
9.	(a)	(b)	(c)	(d)	(e)	51.	(a)	(b)	(c)	(d)	(e)
10.	(a)	(b)	(c)	(d)	(e)	52.	(a)	(b)	(c)	(d)	(e)
11.	(a)	(b)	(c)	(d)	(e)	53.	(a)	(b)	(c)	(d)	(e)
12.	(a)	(b)	(c)	(d)	(e)	54.	(a)	(b)	(c)	(d)	(e)
13.	(a)	(b)	(c)	(d)	(e)	55.	(a)	(b)	(c)	(d)	(e)
14.	(a)	(b)	(c)	(d)	(e)	56.	(a)	(b)	(c)	(d)	(e)
15.	(a)	(b)	(c)	(d)	(e)	57.	(a)	(b)	(c)	(d)	(e)
16.	(a)	(b)	(c)	(d)	(e)	58.	(a)	(b)	(c)	(d)	(e)
17.	(a)	(b)	(c)	(d)	(e)	59.	(a)	(b)	(c)	(d)	(e)
18.	(a)	(b)	(c)	(d)	(e)	60.	(a)	(b)	(c)	(d)	(e)
19.	(a)	(b)	(c)	(d)	(e)	61.	(a)	(b)	(c)	(d)	(e)
20.	(a)	(b)	(c)	(d)	(e)	62.	(a)	(b)	(c)	(d)	(e)
21.	(a)	(b)	(c)	(d)	(e)	63.	(a)	(b)	(c)	(d)	(e)
22.	(a)	(b)	(c)	(d)	(e)	64.	(a)	(b)	(c)	(d)	(e)
23.	(a)	(b)	(c)	(d)	(e)	65.	(a)	(b)	(c)	(d)	(e)
24.	(a)	(b)	(c)	(d)	(e)	66.	(a)	(b)	(c)	(d)	(e)
25.	(a)	(b)	(c)	(d)	(e)	67.	(a)	(b)	(c)	(d)	(e)
26.	(a)	(b)	(c)	(d)	(e)	68.	(a)	(b)	(c)	(d)	(e)
27.	(a)	(b)	(c)	(d)	(e)	69.	(a)	(b)	(c)	(d)	(e)
28.	(a)	(b)	(c)	(d)	(e)	70.	(a)	(b)	(c)	(d)	(e)
29.	(a)	(b)	(c)	(d)	(e)	71.	(a)	(b)	(c)	(d)	(e)
30.	(a)	(b)	(c)	(d)	(e)	72.	(a)	(b)	(c)	(d)	(e)
31.	(a)	(b)	(c)	(d)	(e)	73.	(a)	(b)	(c)	(d)	(e)
32.	(a)	(b)	(c)	(d)	(e)	74.	(a)	(b)	(c)	(d)	(e)
33.	(a)	(b)	(c)	(d)	(e)	75.	(a)	(b)	(c)	(d)	(e)
34.	(a)	(b)	(c)	(d)	(e)	76.	(a)	(b)	(c)	(d)	(e)
35.	(a)	(b)	(c)	(d)	(e)	77.	(a)	(b)	(c)	(d)	(e)
36.	(a)	(b)	(c)	(d)	(e)	78.	(a)	(b)	(c)	(d)	(e)
37.	(a)	(b)	(c)	(d)	(e)	79.	(a)	(b)	(c)	(d)	(e)
38.	(a)	(b)	(c)	(d)	(e)	80.	(a)	(b)	(c)	(d)	(e)
39.	(a)	(b)	(c)	(d)	(e)	81.	(a)	(b)	(c)	(d)	(e)
40.	(a)	(b)	(c)	(d)	(e)	82.	(a)	(b)	(c)	(d)	(e)
41.	(a)	(b)	(c)	(d)	(e)	83.	(a)	(b)	(c)	(d)	(e)
42.	(a)	(b)	(c)	(d)	(e)	84.	(a)	(b)	(c)	(d)	(e)

85.	(a)	(b)	(c)	(d)	(e)
86.	(a)	(b)	(c)	(d)	(e)
87.	(a)	(h)	(r)	(d)	(e)
88.	(a)	(b)	(c)	(d)	(e)
89.	(a)	(b)	(c)	(d)	(e)
90.	(a)	(b)	(c)	(d)	(e)
91.	(a)	(b)	(c)	(d)	(e)
92.	(a)	(b)	(c)	(d)	(e)
93.	(a)	(b)	(c)	(d)	(e)
94.	(a)	(b)	(c)	(d)	(e)
95.	(a)	(b)	(c)	(d)	(e)
96.	(a)	(b)	(c)	(d)	(e)
97.	(a)	(b)	(c)	(d)	(e)
98.	(a)	(b)	(c)	(d)	(e)
99.	(a)	(b)	(c)	(d)	(e)
100.	(a)	(b)	(c)	(d)	(e)
101.	(a)	(b)	(c)	(d)	(e)
102.	(a)	(b)	(c)	(d)	(e)
103.	(a)	(b)	(c)	(d)	(e)
104.	(a)	(b)	(c)	(d)	(e)
105.	(a)	(b)	(c)	(d)	(e)
106.	(a)	(b)	(c)	(d)	(e)
107.	(a)	(b)	(c)	(d)	(e)
108.	(a)	(b)	(c)	(d)	(e)
109.	(a)	(b)	(c)	(d)	(e)
110.	(a)	(b)	(c)	(d)	(e)
111.	(a)	(b)	(c)	(d)	(e)
112.	(a)	(b)	(c)	(d)	(e)
113.	(a)	(b)	(c)	(d)	(e)
114.	(a)	(b)	(c)	(d)	(e)
115.	(a)	(b)	(c)	(d)	(e)
116.	(a)	(b)	(c)	(d)	(e)
117.	(a)	(b)	(c)	(d)	(e)
118.	(a)	(b)	(c)	(d)	(e)
119.	(a)	(b)	(c)	(d)	(e)
120.	(a)	(b)	(c)	(d)	(e)
121.	(a)	(b)	(c)	(d)	(e)
122.	(a)	(b)	(c)	(d)	(e)
123.	(a)	(b)	(c)	(d)	(e)
124.	(a)	(b)	(c)	(d)	(e)
125.	(a)	(b)	(c)	(d)	(e)
126.	(a)	(b)	(c)	(d)	(e)
127.	(a)	(b)	(c)	(d)	(e)
128.	(a)	(b)	(c)	(d)	(e)
129.	(a)	(b)	(c)	(d)	(e)
130.	(a)	(b)	(c)	(d)	(e)
131.	(a)	(b)	(c)	(d)	(e)

132.	(a)	(b)	(c)	(d)	(e)
133.	(a)	(b)	(c)	(d)	(e)
134.	(a)	(h)	(r)	(d)	(e)
135.	(a)	(b)	(c)	(d)	(e)
136.	(a)	(b)	(c)	(d)	(e)
137.	(a)	(b)	(c)	(d)	(e)
138.	(a)	(b)	(c)	(d)	(e)
139.	(a)	(b)	(c)	(d)	(e)
140.	(a)	(b)	(c)	(d)	(e)
141.	(a)	(b)	(c)	(d)	(e)
142.	(a)	(b)	(c)	(d)	(e)
143.	(a)	(b)	(c)	(d)	(e)
144.	(a)	(b)	(c)	(d)	(e)
145.	(a)	(b)	(c)	(d)	(e)
146.	(a)	(b)	(c)	(d)	(e)
147.	(a)	(b)	(c)	(d)	(e)
148.	(a)	(b)	(c)	(d)	(e)
149.	(a)	(b)	(c)	(d)	(e)
150.	(a)	(b)	(c)	(d)	(e)
151.	(a)	(b)	(c)	(d)	(e)
152.	(a)	(b)	(c)	(d)	(e)
153.	(a)	(b)	(c)	(d)	(e)
154.	(a)	(b)	(c)	(d)	(e)
155.	(a)	(b)	(c)	(d)	(e)
156.	(a)	(b)	(c)	(d)	(e)
157.	(a)	(b)	(c)	(d)	(e)
158.	(a)	(b)	(c)	(d)	(e)
159.	(a)	(b)	(c)	(d)	(e)
160.	(a)	(b)	(c)	(d)	(e)
161.	(a)	(b)	(c)	(d)	(e)
162.	(a)	(b)	(c)	(d)	(e)
163.	(a)	(b)	(c)	(d)	(e)
164.	(a)	(b)	(c)	(d)	(e)
165.	(a)	(b)	(c)	(d)	(e)
166.	(a)	(b)	(c)	(d)	(e)
167.	(a)	(b)	(c)	(d)	(e)
168.	(a)	(b)	(c)	(d)	(e)
169.	(a)	(b)	(c)	(d)	(e)
170.	(a)	(b)	(c)	(d)	(e)
171.	(a)	(b)	(c)	(d)	(e)
172.	(a)	(b)	(c)	(d)	(e)
173.	(a)	(b)	(c)	(d)	(e)
174.	(a)	(b)	(c)	(d)	(e)
175.	(a)	(b)	(c)	(d)	(e)
176.	(a)	(b)	(c)	(d)	(e)
177.	(a)	(b)	(c)	(d)	(e)
178.	(a)	(b)	(c)	(d)	(e)

179.	(a)	(b)	(c)	(d)	(e)	**226.**	(a)	(b)	(c)	(d)	(e)
180.	(a)	(b)	(c)	(d)	(e)	**227.**	(a)	(b)	(c)	(d)	(e)
181.	(a)	(b)	(c)	(d)	(e)	**228.**	(a)	(b)	(c)	(d)	(e)
182.	(a)	(b)	(c)	(d)	(e)	**229.**	(a)	(b)	(c)	(d)	(e)
183.	(a)	(b)	(c)	(d)	(e)	**230.**	(a)	(b)	(c)	(d)	(e)
184.	(a)	(b)	(c)	(d)	(e)	**231.**	(a)	(b)	(c)	(d)	(e)
185.	(a)	(b)	(c)	(d)	(e)	**232.**	(a)	(b)	(c)	(d)	(e)
186.	(a)	(h)	(c)	(d)	(e)	**233.**	(a)	(h)	(c)	(d)	(e)
187.	(a)	(b)	(c)	(d)	(e)	**234.**	(a)	(b)	(c)	(d)	(e)
188.	(a)	(b)	(c)	(d)	(e)	**235.**	(a)	(b)	(c)	(d)	(e)
189.	(a)	(b)	(c)	(d)	(e)	**236.**	(a)	(b)	(c)	(d)	(e)
190.	(a)	(b)	(c)	(d)	(e)	**237.**	(a)	(b)	(c)	(d)	(e)
191.	(a)	(b)	(c)	(d)	(e)	**238.**	(a)	(b)	(c)	(d)	(e)
192.	(a)	(b)	(c)	(d)	(e)	**239.**	(a)	(b)	(c)	(d)	(e)
193.	(a)	(b)	(c)	(d)	(e)	**240.**	(a)	(b)	(c)	(d)	(e)
194.	(a)	(b)	(c)	(d)	(e)	**241.**	(a)	(b)	(c)	(d)	(e)
195.	(a)	(b)	(c)	(d)	(e)	**242.**	(a)	(b)	(c)	(d)	(e)
196.	(a)	(b)	(c)	(d)	(e)	**243.**	(a)	(b)	(c)	(d)	(e)
197.	(a)	(b)	(c)	(d)	(e)	**244.**	(a)	(b)	(c)	(d)	(e)
198.	(a)	(b)	(c)	(d)	(e)	**245.**	(a)	(b)	(c)	(d)	(e)
199.	(a)	(b)	(c)	(d)	(e)	**246.**	(a)	(b)	(c)	(d)	(e)
200.	(a)	(b)	(c)	(d)	(e)	**247.**	(a)	(b)	(c)	(d)	(e)
201.	(a)	(b)	(c)	(d)	(e)	**248.**	(a)	(b)	(c)	(d)	(e)
202.	(a)	(b)	(c)	(d)	(e)	**249.**	(a)	(b)	(c)	(d)	(e)
203.	(a)	(b)	(c)	(d)	(e)	**250.**	(a)	(b)	(c)	(d)	(e)
204.	(a)	(b)	(c)	(d)	(e)						
205.	(a)	(b)	(c)	(d)	(e)						
206.	(a)	(b)	(c)	(d)	(e)						
207.	(a)	(b)	(c)	(d)	(e)						
208.	(a)	(b)	(c)	(d)	(e)						
209.	(a)	(b)	(c)	(d)	(e)						
210.	(a)	(b)	(c)	(d)	(e)						
211.	(a)	(b)	(c)	(d)	(e)						
212.	(a)	(b)	(c)	(d)	(e)						
213.	(a)	(b)	(c)	(d)	(e)						
214.	(a)	(b)	(c)	(d)	(e)						
215.	(a)	(b)	(c)	(d)	(e)						
216.	(a)	(b)	(c)	(d)	(e)						
217.	(a)	(b)	(c)	(d)	(e)						
218.	(a)	(b)	(c)	(d)	(e)						
219.	(a)	(b)	(c)	(d)	(e)						
220.	(a)	(b)	(c)	(d)	(e)						
221.	(a)	(b)	(c)	(d)	(e)						
222.	(a)	(b)	(c)	(d)	(e)						
223.	(a)	(b)	(c)	(d)	(e)						
224.	(a)	(b)	(c)	(d)	(e)						
225.	(a)	(b)	(c)	(d)	(e)						

TEST SECTION ONE ANSWER KEY

The page numbers following each answer indicate that subject's reference page within Brady's *Emergency Care*, 5th ed., 1990. If you do not have access to Brady's text, utilize the index of the text you do have to obtain information for review of that subject.

For questions 91 through 139, following each answer is "g/d." This indicates that you should consult the glossary of your EMT text or a medical dictionary.

QUESTION	ANSWER	PAGE REFERENCE *Emergency Care* 5th edition	
1.	(d)	page 12	EMT responsibilities
2.	(d)	page 14	assessment
3.	(d)	page 17	negligence
4.	(b)	page 17	documentation
5.	(e)	page 17	standard of care
6.	(e)	page 18	actual consent
7.	(b)	page 18	abandonment
8.	(a)	page 19	implied consent
9.	(a)	page 19	implied consent
10.	(c)	page 19	consent of a minor
11.	(c)	page 19	Good Samaritan Laws
12.	(d)	page 32	lateral
13.	(b)	page 32	extension
14.	(e)	page 32	medial
15.	(c)	page 32	flexion
16.	(a)	page 33	anatomy
17.	(b)	page 33	physiology
18.	(e)	page 33	anatomical position
19.	(e)	page 33	lateral
20.	(c)	page 33	midline
21.	(d)	page 33	inferior
22.	(a)	page 33	superior
23.	(b)	page 33	medial
24.	(e)	page 33	distal
25.	(b)	page 33	anterior
26.	(a)	page 33	proximal
27.	(d)	page 33	posterior
28.	(c)	page 33	anterior
29.	(e)	page 34	supine
30.	(a)	page 34	prone
31.	(b)	page 34	lateral recumbent

QUESTION	ANSWER	PAGE REFERENCE *Emergency Care* *5th edition*	
32.	(c)	page 34	abduction
33.	(a)	page 34	adduction
34.	(b)	page 36	skull
35.	(e)	page 36	spinal column
36.	(b)	page 37	sacrum
37.	(a)	page 37	thoracic spine
38.	(d)	page 37	cervical spine
39.	(e)	page 37	coccyx
40.	(c)	page 37	lumbar spine
41.	(e)	page 37	diaphragm
42.	(c)	page 38	liver
43.	(b)	page 38	intestines
44.	(d)	page 38	spleen
45.	(e)	page 38	appendix
46.	(d)	page 62	carotid pulse
47.	(a)	page 62	radial pulse
48.	(c)	page 62	brachial pulse
49.	(b)	page 62	femoral pulse
50.	(e)	page 62	pedal pulse
51.	(a)	page 62	auscultation
52.	(c)	page 62	palpation
53.	(d)	page 70	primary survey
54.	(b)	page 72	jaw thrust
55.	(a)	page 73	vital signs
56.	(c)	page 73	primary survey
57.	(b)	page 75	secondary survey
58.	(a)	page 79	Glasgow Coma Scale
59.	(e)	page 82	signs and symptoms
60.	(d)	page 82	signs and symptoms
61.	(d)	page 83	cyanosis
62.	(e)	page 83	jaundice
63.	(b)	page 83	skin color
64.	(a)	page 83	jaundice
65.	(d)	page 83	skin color
66.	(b)	page 85	pulse rates
67.	(c)	page 85	pulse rates
68.	(b)	page 87	respiratory rates
69.	(e)	page 87	respiratory rates
70.	(c)	page 87	respiratory rates
71.	(a)	page 88	diastolic blood pressure
72.	(d)	page 88	systolic blood pressure
73.	(e)	page 88	auscultated blood pressure
74.	(c)	page 88	auscultated blood pressure
75.	(d)	page 88	palpated blood pressure
76.	(e)	page 88	palpated blood pressure

PAGE REFERENCE
Emergency Care
5th edition

QUESTION	ANSWER		
77.	(c)	page 88	palpated blood pressure
78.	(c)	page 516	triage
79.	(e)	page 516	triage
80.	(d)	page 516	triage
81.	(c)	page 516	triage
82.	(a)	page 542	ambulance operation
83.	(d)	page 544	hydroplaning
84.	(c)	page 546	ambulance operation
85.	(d)	page 552	ambulance operation
86.	(a)	page 556	ambulance operation
87.	(e)	page 565	lifting and moving
88.	(c)	page 565	lifting and moving
89.	(d)	page 568	lifting and moving
90.	(e)	page 605	documentation
91.	(d)	g/d	hematoma
92.	(a)	g/d	hemorrhage
93.	(c)	g/d	hematuria
94.	(a)	g/d	hemorrhage
95.	(b)	g/d	hematemesis
96.	(e)	g/d	hemoptysis
97.	(c)	g/d	hyperextension
98.	(a)	g/d	hyperflexion
99.	(d)	g/d	hyperthermia
100.	(e)	g/d	hypothermia
101.	(a)	g/d	hyperventilation
102.	(c)	g/d	dyspnea
103.	(d)	g/d	tachypnea
104.	(e)	g/d	hyperpnea
105.	(a)	g/d	inspiration/inhalation
106.	(b)	g/d	expiration/exhalation
107.	(c)	g/d	-ectomy
108.	(a)	g/d	-itis
109.	(e)	g/d	laceration
110.	(b)	g/d	incision
111.	(b)	g/d	contusion
112.	(e)	g/d	abrasion
113.	(a)	g/d	epistaxis
114.	(d)	g/d	emesis
115.	(d)	g/d	syncope
116.	(c)	g/d	nausea
117.	(d)	g/d	vertigo
118.	(b)	g/d	febrile
119.	(d)	g/d	a-
120.	(c)	g/d	acute
121.	(a)	g/d	chronic

QUESTION	ANSWER	PAGE REFERENCE *Emergency Care* *5th edition*	
122.	(c)	g/d	paralysis
123.	(d)	g/d	hemiplegia
124.	(b)	g/d	paraplegia
125.	(e)	g/d	quadriplegia
126.	(a)	g/d	hypertensive
127.	(b)	g/d	hypotensive
128.	(c)	g/d	referred pain
129.	(a)	g/d	radiation of pain
130.	(d)	g/d	tachycardia
131.	(b)	g/d	bradycardia
132.	(b)	g/d	bilateral
133.	(c)	g/d	unilateral
134.	(e)	g/d	aspiration
135.	(c)	g/d	apnea
136.	(e)	g/d	hypoxia
137.	(d)	g/d	penetrating wound
138.	(c)	g/d	perforating wound
139.	(b)	g/d	perfusion

TEST SECTION TWO ANSWER KEY

The page numbers following each answer indicate that subject's reference page within Brady's *Emergency Care*, 5th ed., 1990. If you do not have access to Brady's text, utilize the index of the text you do have to obtain information for review of that subject.

Following some answers is "g/d." This indicates that you should consult the glossary of your EMT text or a medical dictionary.

QUESTION	ANSWER	PAGE REFERENCE *Emergency Care* 5th edition	
1.	(b)	page 113	carbon dioxide
2.	(a)	page 113	gas exchange
3.	(b)	page 113	gas exchange
4.	(d)	page 113	gas exchange
5.	(e)	page 113	gas exchange
6.	(d)	page 114	biological death
7.	(a)	page 114	clinical death
8.	(c)	page 114	brain death
9.	(e)	pages 52, 114	pleura
10.	(b)	pages 52, 114	diaphragm
11.	(c)	pages 52, 114	alveoli
12.	(c)	pages 52, 114	pharynx
13.	(e)	pages 52, 114	bronchi
14.	(d)	pages 52, 114	trachea
15.	(b)	pages 52, 114	epiglottis
16.	(a)	pages 52, 114	larynx
17.	(d)	page 114	primary airway
18.	(b)	page 114	secondary airway
19.	(d)	page 115	respiration
20.	(b)	page 115	respiration
21.	(c)	page 115	pleura function
22.	(a)	page 115	respiratory center
23.	(a)	page 115	increased blood levels of carbon dioxide
24.	(a)	page 115	decreased blood levels of oxygen
25.	(d)	page 116	adequate/inadequate breathing
26.	(c)	page 116	adult respiratory rate
27.	(d)	page 116	cyanosis
28.	(c)	page 143	cardiac arrest
29.	(a)	page 116	respiratory arrest
30.	(a)	page 116	pulmonary resuscitation
31.	(c)	page 141	cardiopulmonary arrest
32.	(c)	page 116	abdominal breathing
33.	(b)	page 116	inadequate breathing

PAGE REFERENCE

QUESTION	ANSWER	*Emergency Care* *5th edition*	
34.	(b)	page 116	inadequate breathing
35.	(e)	page 117	airway obstruction
36.	(b)	page 119	head-tilt chin-lift
37.	(e)	page 119	airway maneuvers
38.	(c)	page 119	modified jaw thrust
39.	(b)	page 119	head-tilt chin-lift
40.	(e)	page 120	artificial respirations
41.	(e)	page 120	oxygen content of room air
42.	(d)	page 120	oxygen content of expired air
43.	(a)	page 120	pulmonary resuscitation
44.	(c)	page 120	determining breathlessness
45.	(e)	page 121	rescue breathing
46.	(d)	page 121	adequate ventilation
47.	(a)	page 121	ventilation interference
48.	(b)	page 121	artificial respiration—adult rate
49.	(c)	page 122	artificial respiration—child rate
50.	(d)	page 122	artificial respiration—infant rate
51.	(b)	page 122	mouth-to-nose respirations
52.	(e)	page 122	mouth-to-nose respirations
53.	(e)	page 122	artificial respirations—infant/child
54.	(c)	page 122	laryngectomy patient
55.	(d)	page 122	stoma
56.	(e)	page 124	stoma ventilations
57.	(a)	page 124	gastric distention
58.	(b)	page 125	airway obstruction
59.	(d)	page 126	skin color assessment
60.	(e)	page 126	partial airway obstruction
61.	(c)	page 126	complete airway obstruction
62.	(c)	pages 127, 130	obstructed airway care
63.	(b)	page 128	chest thrusts
64.	(a)	page 129	finger sweeps
65.	(c)	page 131	obstructed airway care
66.	(b)	page 131	obstructed airway care
67.	(a)	page 131	obstructed airway care
68.	(e)	page 131	obstructed airway care
69.	(c)	page 132	obstructed airway care
70.	(c)	page 132	obstructed airway care
71.	(a)	page 132	obstructed airway care
72.	(c)	page 139	the heart
73.	(b)	page 139	the heart
74.	(c)	page 139	the heart
75.	(a)	page 139	the heart
76.	(e)	page 139	the heart
77.	(d)	page 139	the heart
78.	(b)	page 139	the heart

QUESTION	ANSWER	PAGE REFERENCE *Emergency Care* 5th edition	
79.	(c)	page 139	arteries
80.	(a)	page 139	veins
81.	(e)	page 139	capillaries
82.	(d)	page 141	artificial circulation
83.	(c)	page 142	CPR effectiveness
84.	(e)	page 143	CPR performance
85.	(e)	page 143	determination of pulselessness
86.	(b)	page 143	CPR performance
87.	(d)	page 143	CPR performance
88.	(d)	page 143	CPR performance
89.	(d)	page 143	CPR performance
90.	(a)	page 144	CPR performance
91.	(b)	page 144	hand placement—adult
92.	(d)	page 145	depth of compression—adult
93.	(c)	page 155	depth of compression—child
94.	(b)	page 155	depth of compression—infant
95.	(b)	page 155	age range of child
96.	(c)	page 155	age range of infant
97.	(d)	page 145	depth of compression-adult
98.	(b)	page 145	compression rate-adult
99.	(b)	page 156	compression rate-child
100.	(c)	page 156	compression rate-infant
101.	(b)	page 145	compression rate-adult
102.	(e)	page 144	compression site-adult
103.	(a)	page 146	pulse checks
104.	(c)	page 146	effective CPR
105.	(d)	page 147	xyphoid process
106.	(d)	page 147	CPR complications
107.	(d)	page 147	CPR complications
108.	(b)	page 147	CPR complications
109.	(c)	page 147	CPR complications
110.	(d)	page 148	CPR and terminal illness
111.	(a)	page 148	terminating CPR
112.	(a)	page 149	adult CPR
113.	(e)	page 149	adult CPR
114.	(e)	page 156	chiLd CPR
115.	(e)	page 156	child CPR
116.	(e)	page 156	infant CPR
117.	(e)	page 156	infant CPR
118.	(b)	page 149	interuption of CPR
119.	(b)	page 149	two-rescuer CPR
120.	(c)	page 149	pulse checks
121.	(c)	page 152	two-rescuer CPR
122.	(a)	page 155	infant pulse check site

		PAGE REFERENCE	
QUESTION	**ANSWER**	*Emergency Care* *5th edition*	
123.	(c)	page 155	child pulse check site
124.	(b)	page 155	infant compression site
125.	(a)	page 155	child compression site
126.	(d)	page 164	airway adjuncts
127.	(b)	page 166	nasopharyngeal airway
128.	(b)	page 166	nasopharyngeal airway
129.	(a)	page 164	oropharyngeal airway
130.	(a)	page 164	oropharyngeal airway
131.	(b)	page 166	nasopharyngeal airway
132.	(a)	page 164	oropharyngeal airway
133.	(b)	page 166	nasopharyngeal airway
134.	(b)	page 166	nasopharyngeal airway
135.	(d)	page 164	airway adjuncts
136.	(e)	page 164	oropharyngeal airway
137.	(a)	page 166	nasopharyngeal airway
138.	(e)	page 166	nasopharyngeal airway
139.	(c)	page 166	airway lubricants
140.	(b)	page 164	oropharyngeal airway
141.	(d)	page 168	rigid suction
142.	(e)	page 168	suction
143.	(d)	page 168	suction
144.	(c)	page 168	suction
145.	(a)	page 168	suction
146.	(e)	page 169	suction
147.	(b)	page 170	pocket mask
148.	(d)	page 170	pocket mask
149.	(e)	page 171	pocket mask
150.	(a)	page 171	bag-valve-mask device
151.	(d)	page 171	bag-valve-mask device
152.	(a)	page 173	oxygen
153.	(c)	page 174	hypoxic
154.	(d)	g/d	hypoxemia
155.	(b)	page 173	hypoxia
156.	(a)	page 174	anoxia
157.	(e)	pages 173, 174	oxygen
158.	(d)	page 174	oxygen side effects
159.	(a)	page 176	oxygen cylinders
160.	(b)	page 176	oxygen cylinders
161.	(e)	page 176	oxygen cylinders
162.	(c)	page 176	oxygen cylinders
163.	(d)	page 176	oxygen cylinders
164.	(b)	page 181	oxygen flow rates
165.	(c)	page 181	oxygen flow rates
166.	(c)	page 181	oxygen flow rates

QUESTION	ANSWER	PAGE REFERENCE *Emergency Care* *5th edition*	
167.	(a)	page 181	oxygen flow rates
168.	(e)	page 181	oxygen flow rates
169.	(a)	page 181	oxygen delivery concentrations
170.	(d)	page 181	oxygen delivery concentrations
171.	(d)	page 181	oxygen delivery concentrations
172.	(b)	page 181	oxygen delivery concentrations
173.	(e)	page 181	oxygen delivery concentrations
174.	(b)	pages 181-183	oxygen administration
175.	(b)	page 183	BVM device and demand valve resuscitator
176.	(c)	page 371	congenital anomaly
177.	(e)	page 372	acute
178.	(c)	page 372	chronic
179.	(a)	page 372	episodic
180.	(e)	page 372	acute
181.	(b)	page 373	poison
182.	(d)	page 373	venom
183.	(a)	page 373	toxin
184.	(b)	page 374	systemic reaction
185.	(c)	g/d	localized reaction
186.	(b)	page 374	systemic poisons
187.	(c)	page 374	ingested poisons
188.	(a)	page 374	inhaled poisons
189.	(e)	page 374	absorbed poisons
190.	(d)	page 374	injected poisons
191.	(c)	page 376	treatment of ingested poisons
192.	(d)	page 376	signs and symptoms of ingested poisons
193.	(e)	page 376	induced vomiting
194.	(e)	page 376	induced vomiting
195.	(c)	page 376	antiemetics
196.	(a)	page 376	plant ingestions
197.	(e)	page 378	treatment of inhaled poisons
198.	(c)	page 379	treatment of absorbed poisons
199.	(c)	page 379	black widow spider
200.	(a)	page 379	brown recluse spider
201.	(d)	page 379	spider bites
202.	(b)	page 380	treatment of stings
203.	(b)	page 380	United States snakes
204.	(a)	page 380	types of poisonous snakes
205.	(a)	page 380	dangerous snakes
206.	(e)	page 380	pit vipers
207.	(a)	page 380	coral snakes
208.	(b)	page 380	pit vipers
209.	(e)	page 380	coral snakes
210.	(a)	page 380	nonpoisonous snakes

PAGE REFERENCE
Emergency Care
5th edition

QUESTION	ANSWER		
211.	(d)	page 381	treatment of snake bites
212.	(c)	page 386	the heart pacemaker
213.	(d)	page 386	coronary arteries
214.	(c)	page 386	myocardium
215.	(c)	page 386	atherosclerosis
216.	(d)	page 386	arteriosclerosis
217.	(b)	page 387	aneurism
218.	(c)	page 386	plaque
219.	(e)	page 387	embolus
220.	(b)	page 387	emboli
221.	(d)	page 387	thrombus
222.	(a)	page 387	occlusion
223.	(b)	page 388	infarction
224.	(a)	page 388	angina pectoris
225.	(b)	page 388	acute myocardial infarction
226.	(c)	page 388	nitroglycerin
227.	(d)	page 388	nitroglycerin
228.	(e)	page 388	nitroglycerin
229.	(d)	page 388	acute myocardial infarction
230.	(e)	page 390	acute myocardial infarction
231.	(d)	page 392	congestive heart failure
232.	(c)	page 392	congestive heart failure
233.	(b)	page 393	pulmonary edema
234.	(e)	page 393	pedal edema/peripheral edema
235.	(a)	page 393	peripheral edema
236.	(d)	page 393	ascities
237.	(e)	pages 388-394	AMI, CHF, angina
238.	(a)	pages 388-394	acute myocardial infarction
239.	(e)	pages 388-394	chest pain
240.	(c)	pages 388-394	congestive heart failure
241.	(e)	pages 388-394	irregular pulse
242.	(d)	pages 388-394	chest pain
243.	(e)	pages 388-394	blood pressure
244.	(b)	pages 388-394	angina
245.	(e)	pages 388-394	hypotension
246.	(e)	pages 388-394	chest pain
247.	(e)	page 389	treatment of angina
248.	(d)	page 391	treatment of acute myocardial infarction
249.	(a)	page 393	treatment of congestive heart failure
250.	(b)	page 393	cerebrovascular accident
251.	(b)	page 394	cerebrovascular accident
252.	(a)	page 394	cerebrovascular accident
253.	(c)	page 394	treatment of cerebrovascular accident
254.	(e)	pages 394, 399	dyspnea

		PAGE REFERENCE	
QUESTION	**ANSWER**	*Emergency Care* *5th edition*	
255.	(c)	page 394	dyspnea
256.	(b)	page 394	aphasia
257.	(e)	page 399	tachypnea
258.	(d)	page 399	apnea
259.	(a)	page 396	asphyxia
260.	(b)	page 397	primary respiratory stimulus
261.	(d)	page 397	secondary respiratory stimulus
262.	(d)	pages 397, 175	COPD primary respiratory stimulus
263.	(b)	pages 397, 398	chronic bronchitis
264.	(c)	pages 397, 398	emphysema
265.	(a)	pages 397, 398	asthma
266.	(d)	page 398	hypoxic drive
267.	(d)	page 398	treatment of emphysema
268.	(d)	page 398	treatment of chronic bronchitis
269.	(c)	page 398	treatment of asthma
270.	(a)	page 398	hyperventilation
271.	(d)	page 399	hyperventilation
272.	(a)	page 399	spontaneous pneumothorax

TEST SECTION THREE ANSWER KEY

The page numbers following each answer indicate that subject's reference page within Brady's *Emergency Care*, 5th ed., 1990. If you do not have access to Brady's text, utilize the index of the text you do have to obtain information for review of that subject.

		PAGE REFERENCE	
QUESTION	ANSWER	*Emergency Care* 5th edition	
1.	(d)	page 402	acute abdomen
2.	(c)	page 403	diabetes
3.	(b)	pages 403-405	insulin shock
4.	(a)	pages 403-405	diabetic coma
5.	(b)	pages 403-405	hypoglycemia
6.	(d)	pages 403-405	diabetes
7.	(a)	pages 403-405	hyperglycemia
8.	(b)	pages 403-405	hyperglycemia
9.	(b)	pages 403-405	hypoglycemia
10.	(b)	pages 403-405	hypoglycemia
11.	(d)	pages 403-405	diabetes
12.	(a)	pages 403-405	hyperglycemia
13.	(a)	pages 403-405	hyperglycemia
14.	(e)	pages 403-405	seizures
15.	(d)	pages 403-405	diabetes
16.	(a)	pages 403-405	hyperglycemia
17.	(c)	pages 403-405	hypoglycemia
18.	(c)	pages 403-405	hypoglycemia
19.	(a)	pages 403-405	hyperglycemia
20.	(d)	page 404	treatment of diabetes
21.	(b)	page 406	convulsion
22.	(a)	page 406	seizure
23.	(a)	page 407	status epilepticus
24.	(d)	page 406	causes of convulsions
25.	(e)	page 406	seizures
26.	(b)	page 406	grand mal seizures
27.	(b)	page 406	grand mal seizures
28.	(e)	page 406	seizure
29.	(e)	page 406	treatment of seizures
30.	(c)	page 407	acute abdominal distress
31.	(e)	page 408	acute abdominal distress
32.	(d)	page 408	acute abdominal distress
33.	(c)	page 409	universal precautions
34.	(c)	page 409	airborne droplet disease transmission

QUESTION	ANSWER	PAGE REFERENCE *Emergency Care* 5th edition	
35.	(a)	page 409	direct contact disease transmission
36.	(b)	page 409	indirect contact disease transmission
37.	(a)	page 411	alcohol
38.	(d)	page 411	alcohol intoxication
39.	(b)	page 411	alcohol intoxication
40.	(a)	page 411	treatment of alcohol intoxication
41.	(e)	page 411	delirium tremens
42.	(d)	page 411	delirium tremens
43.	(c)	page 411	alcohol withdrawal
44.	(c)	page 413	amphetamine abuse
45.	(b)	page 413	CNS depressants
46.	(c)	page 413	hallucinogens
47.	(a)	page 413	CNS stimulants
48.	(d)	pages 413, 414	barbiturate abuse
49.	(e)	pages 413, 414	tranquilizer abuse
50.	(a)	page 414	opiate abuse
51.	(d)	page 414	inhalant abuse
52.	(e)	page 414	hallucinogen abuse
53.	(b)	page 418	infant age range
54.	(d)	page 418	child age range
55.	(d)	pages 424, 425	pediatric trauma
56.	(b)	page 426	child abuse
57.	(d)	page 428	pediatric sexual assault
58.	(e)	page 428	pediatric fever
59.	(b)	page 429	epiglottitis
60.	(a)	page 429	croup
61.	(d)	page 429	treatment of epiglottitis and croup
62.	(b)	page 429	treatment of epiglottitis
63.	(b)	page 429	treatment of epiglottitis
64.	(e)	page 430	bronchitis, bronchiolitis, asthma
65.	(c)	page 430	pediatric asthma
66.	(e)	page 430	tx of bronchitis/bronchiolitis/asthma
67.	(d)	page 430	pediatric poisonings
68.	(a)	page 431	Sudden Infant Death Syndrome
69.	(e)	page 193	leukocytes
70.	(d)	page 193	red blood cells
71.	(e)	page 193	white blood cells
72.	(b)	page 193	platelets
73.	(d)	page 193	erythrocytes
74.	(a)	page 193	plasma
75.	(b)	page 193	average adult blood volume
76.	(c)	page 193	adult shock blood loss
77.	(b)	page 193	child shock blood loss
78.	(a)	pages 139, 194	arteries

		PAGE REFERENCE	
QUESTION	**ANSWER**	*Emergency Care*	
		5th edition	
79.	(c)	pages 139, 194	veins
80.	(b)	pages 139, 194	capillaries
81.	(e)	pages 140, 194	pulmonary arteries
82.	(d)	pages 140, 194	pulmonary veins
83.	(d)	page 194	perfusion
84.	(b)	page 194	arterial bleeding
85.	(a)	page 194	venous bleeding
86.	(c)	page 194	capillary bleeding
87.	(c)	pages 195-197	direct pressure
88.	(a)	page 197	elevation and pressure points
89.	(a)	page 198	tourniquets
90.	(e)	page 200	internal bleeding
91.	(c)	page 201	signs and symptoms of internal bleeding
92.	(a)	page 202	treatment of internal bleeding
93.	(d)	page 342	epistaxis
94.	(a)	page 202	shock
95.	(e)	page 202	shock
96.	(d)	page 203	metabolic shock
97.	(a)	page 203	septic shock
98.	(e)	page 203	psychogenic shock
99.	(c)	page 203	anaphylactic shock
100.	(b)	page 203	hypovolemic shock
101.	(d)	page 203	psychogenic shock
102.	(e)	page 203	cardiogenic shock
103.	(c)	page 203	neurogenic shock
104.	(b)	page 203	respiratory shock
105.	(a)	page 203	hemorrhagic shock
106.	(e)	page 204	cardiogenic shock
107.	(c)	page 204	signs and symptoms of shock
108.	(b)	page 204	signs and symptoms of shock
109.	(a)	page 204	signs and symptoms of shock
110.	(b)	page 205	capillary refill
111.	(c)	page 371	diaphoresis
112.	(b)	page 205	treatment of shock
113.	(d)	page 206	treatment of shock
114.	(b)	page 207	anaphylactic shock
115.	(d)	page 208	anaphylactic shock
116.	(d)	page 208	signs and symptoms of anaphylactic shock
117.	(e)	page 209	treatment of anaphylactic shock
118.	(b)	page 211	PASG
119.	(c)	page 212	anti-shock garment
120.	(d)	pages 212, 213	MAST
121.	(d)	page 212	MAST
122.	(d)	page 213	MAST

		PAGE REFERENCE	
QUESTION	**ANSWER**	*Emergency Care* *5th edition*	
123.	(d)	page 213	MAST
124.	(b)	page 218	skin
125.	(b)	page 219	dermis
126.	(c)	page 219	epidermis
127.	(a)	page 219	subcutaneous tissuc
128.	(c)	page 219	epidermis
129.	(a)	page 219	subcutaneous tissue
130.	(b)	page 219	dermis
131.	(e)	page 220	contusion
132.	(b)	page 220	ecchymosis
133.	(c)	page 221	abrasion
134.	(e)	page 222	perforating puncture wound
135.	(c)	page 222	penetrating puncture wound
136.	(b)	page 223	avulsion
137.	(a)	page 223	amputation
138.	(e)	pages 221, 223	blunt force injury
139.	(e)	pages 221, 223	crushing force injury
140.	(c)	page 224	dressings and bandages
141.	(b)	page 225	occlusive dressings
142.	(d)	page 228	impaled objects
143.	(b)	page 230	treatment of avulsion and amputation
144.	(e)	page 230	treatment of avulsion and amputation
145.	(a)	page 230	evisceration
146.	(c)	pages 230, 362	treatment of evisceration
147.	(e)	page 238	cardiac muscle
148.	(b)	page 238	involuntary muscle
149.	(b)	page 238	involuntary muscle
150.	(a)	page 238	voluntary muscle
151.	(d)	page 238	diaphragm muscle
152.	(c)	page 238	skeleton
153.	(a)	page 239	bones
154.	(c)	page 239	bones
155.	(c)	page 240	axial skeleton
156.	(d)	page 240	appendicular skeleton
157.	(c)	page 240	thoracic cavity
158.	(e)	page 243	scapula
159.	(d)	page 243	radius
160.	(c)	page 243	humerus
161.	(b)	page 243	clavicle
162.	(a)	page 243	ulna
163.	(a)	page 244	patella
164.	(e)	page 244	sacrum
165.	(c)	page 244	femur
166.	(c)	page 244	femur
167.	(b)	page 244	tibia

QUESTION	ANSWER	PAGE REFERENCE *Emergency Care* 5th edition	
168.	(d)	page 244	fibula
169.	(c)	page 243	carpals
170.	(d)	page 243	metacarpals
171.	(e)	page 243	phalanges
172.	(a)	page 244	tarsals
173.	(b)	page 244	metarsals
174.	(e)	page 244	phalanges
175.	(a)	page 245	fractures
176.	(c)	page 246	dislocations
177.	(d)	page 247	sprains
178.	(c)	page 245	greenstick fracture
179.	(a)	page 245	transverse fracture
180.	(e)	page 245	oblique fracture
181.	(d)	page 246	impacted fracture
182.	(b)	page 246	comminuted fracture
183.	(e)	page 247	fracture, dislocation, sprain
184.	(d)	page 247	fracture, dislocation
185.	(a)	page 247	fracture
186.	(a)	page 247	fracture
187.	(c)	page 247	crepitus
188.	(e)	page 248	fracture
189.	(e)	page 254	splinting
190.	(c)	page 252	splinting
191.	(b)	pages 250, 253	treatment of angulated fracture
192.	(d)	pages 250, 256	splinting
193.	(e)	page 257	upper extremity injury
194.	(a)	pages 257-264	upper extremity splinting
195.	(b)	page 270	ilium
196.	(c)	page 270	iliac crests
197.	(a)	page 270	ischium
198.	(d)	page 270	sacrum
199.	(e)	page 270	pubic bones
200.	(e)	page 271	posterior tibial pulse
201.	(b)	page 271	dorsalis pedis pulse
202.	(b)	page 271	dorsalis pedis pulse
203.	(d)	page 273	pelvic fractures
204.	(e)	page 276	femur fracture
205.	(e)	page 276	femur fracture
206.	(a)	page 274	treatment of pelvic fracture
207.	(e)	page 274	hip dislocation vs. fracture
208.	(d)	page 274	hip dislocation vs. fracture
209.	(b)	page 274	hip dislocation vs. fracture
210.	(b)	page 274	posterior hip dislocation
211.	(b)	page 274	sciatic nerve
212.	(c)	page 274	hip fracture

QUESTION	ANSWER	PAGE REFERENCE *Emergency Care* 5th edition	
213.	(a)	page 274	treatment of hip fracture/dislocation
214.	(c)	page 276	femur fracture
215.	(e)	pages 273,276	knee dislocation/fracture
216.	(c)	pages 480,483	evaporation heat loss
217.	(e)	pages 480,483	radiation heat loss
218.	(b)	pages 480,483	convection heat loss
219.	(a)	pages 480,483	conduction heat loss
220.	(d)	pages 480,483	respiration heat loss
221.	(b)	pages 481,482	heat exhaustion
222.	(a)	pages 480,483	heat cramps
223.	(e)	pages 480,483	heat exhaustion/stroke
224.	(c)	pages 480,483	heat stroke
225.	(a)	pages 480,483	heat cramps
226.	(e)	pages 480,483	heat injuries
227.	(a)	pages 480,483	heat cramps
228.	(e)	pages 480,483	heat injuries
229.	(b)	pages 480,483	heat exhaustion
230.	(c)	pages 480,483	heat stroke
231.	(d)	pages 480,483	heat cramps/exhaustion
232.	(e)	pages 480,483	heat exhaustion/stroke
233.	(c)	pages 480,483	heat stroke
234.	(a)	pages 480,483	treatment of heat cramps
235.	(d)	pages 480,483	treatment of heat exhaustion
236.	(c)	pages 480,483	treatment of heat stroke
237.	(d)	page 483	hypothermia
238.	(c)	page 483	hypothermia
239.	(e)	page 483	deep frostbite
240.	(a)	page 483	frostnip
241.	(d)	page 483	superficial frostbite
242.	(a)	page 484	treatment of frostnip
243.	(e)	page 484	treatment of frostbite
244.	(c)	page 484	treatment of frostbite
245.	(d)	page 483	shivering
246.	(e)	page 485	signs and symptoms of hypothermia
247.	(a)	page 485	signs and symptoms of hypothermia
248.	(c)	page 486	treatment of hypothermia
249.	(d)	page 486	treatment of hypothermia
250.	(a)	page 489	near-drowning
251.	(a)	page 489	near-drowning
252.	(c)	pages 490, 492	near-drowning
253.	(e)	pages 195, 495	air embolism
254.	(b)	page 495	signs and symptoms of air embolism
255.	(d)	page 495	decompression sickness
256.	(e)	page 495	signs/symptoms of decompression sickness
257.	(d)	page 496	tx of air embolism/decompression sickness

TEST SECTION FOUR ANSWER KEY

The page numbers following each answer indicate that subject's reference page within Brady's *Emergency Care*, 5th ed., 1990. If you do not have access to Brady's text, utilize the index of the text you do have to obtain information for review of that subject.

Following some answers is "g/d." This indicates that you should consult the glossary of your EMT text or a medical dictionary.

QUESTION	ANSWER	PAGE REFERENCE *Emergency Care* 5th edition	
1.	(b)	page 296	axial skeleton
2.	(c)	page 296	rib cage
3.	(e)	page 297	thoracic spine
4.	(b)	page 297	lumbar spine
5.	(b)	page 297	sacrum
6.	(c)	page 297	cervical spine
7.	(a)	page 297	coccyx
8.	(c)	page 297	mandible
9.	(e)	page 297	sternum
10.	(a)	page 297	zygomatic bone
11.	(e)	page 297	the nervous system
12.	(d)	page 297	central nervous system
13.	(c)	page 297	peripheral nervous system
14.	(c)	page 297	sensory nerves
15.	(d)	page 297	motor nerves
16.	(e)	page 298	autonomic nervous system
17.	(b)	page 298	the brain
18.	(e)	page 299	skull fracture
19.	(a)	page 299	skull fracture
20.	(e)	page 299	basal skull fracture
21.	(c)	page 299	depressed skull fracture
22.	(b)	page 299	comminuted skull fracture
23.	(a)	page 299	linear skull fracture
24.	(d)	page 299	penetrated skull
25.	(b)	page 299	cerebral concussion
26.	(a)	page 299	cerebral contusion
27.	(c)	page 299	cerebral hematoma
28.	(c)	page 299	cerebral concussion
29.	(e)	page 299	cerebral contusion
30.	(c)	page 299	amnesia
31.	(a)	page 299	facial fracture
32.	(b)	page 299	subdural hematoma
33.	(a)	page 300	epidural hematoma

QUESTION	ANSWER	PAGE REFERENCE *Emergency Care* 5th edition	
34.	(c)	page 300	intracerebral hematoma
35.	(e)	page 300	Battle's sign
36.	(d)	page 300	raccoon's sign
37.	(c)	page 300	skull fracture
38.	(d)	page 300	raccoon's eyes
39.	(b)	page 301	cerebrospinal fluid
40.	(e)	page 301	cerebrospinal fluid
41.	(a)	page 302	skull fracture care
42.	(b)	page 302	increased intercrainial pressure
43.	(a)	page 303	Glasgow Coma Scale
44.	(e)	page 303	reporting verbal responses
45.	(c)	page 303	oxygen delivery
46.	(e)	pages 302, 304	head injury care
47.	(a)	page 305	facial fractures
48.	(e)	page 305	impaled skull
49.	(b)	page 306	helmets
50.	(e)	page 306	spine injury
51.	(d)	page 308	spine injury
52.	(d)	page 309	spine injury
53.	(d)	page 311	unconscious trauma patient
54.	(a)	page 313	spinal immobilization
55.	(c)	page 328	face and scalp injury
56.	(a)	page 328	scalp wounds
57.	(d)	page 330	facial trauma care
58.	(a)	page 331	impaled cheek
59.	(b)	page 332	aqueous humor
60.	(c)	page 332	vitreous humor
61.	(a)	page 332	aqueous humor
62.	(e)	page 332	vitreous humor
63.	(c)	page 332	sclera
64.	(a)	page 332	iris
65.	(d)	page 332	conjunctiva
66.	(b)	page 332	cornea
67.	(e)	page 332	lens
68.	(d)	page 332	pupil size
69.	(b)	page 332	pupil size
70.	(e)	page 333	eye care
71.	(a)	page 334	sympathetic eye movement
72.	(a)	page 336	chemical burns to the eye
73.	(c)	page 336	burns to eyelids
74.	(c)	page 336	light burns to the eyes
75.	(c)	page 336	care of impaled eye
76.	(b)	page 337	contact lenses
77.	(b)	page 337	avulsed eye
78.	(c)	page 337	care for avulsed eye

		PAGE REFERENCE	
QUESTION	**ANSWER**	*Emergency Care* 5th edition	
79.	(d)	page 339	the ear
80.	(d)	page 341	ear obstruction
81.	(e)	page 341	obstructed nose
82.	(e)	page 342	nosebleed (epistaxis)
83.	(a)	page 343	avulsed tooth
84.	(a)	page 343	neck trauma
85.	(e)	page 344	neck trauma
86.	(c)	page 344	neck trauma
87.	(b)	page 345	neck trauma
88.	(d)	page 240	chest structure
89.	(d)	page 350	chest trauma
90.	(b)	page 350	chest compression injury
91.	(a)	page 352	signs and symptoms of chest injury
92.	(c)	page 352	subcutaneous emphysema
93.	(c)	page 352	sucking chest wound
94.	(e)	page 352	pneumothorax
95.	(d)	pages 352, 399	pneumothorax
96.	(b)	page 352	pneumothorax
97.	(a)	page 352	occlusive dressing
98.	(d)	pages 354, 399	tension pneumothorax
99.	(d)	page 354	tension pneumothorax
100.	(e)	page 354	tension pneumothorax
101.	(b)	page 355	impaled chest
102.	(d)	page 356	rib fracture
103.	(c)	page 357	chest injury
104.	(c)	page 357	flail chest
105.	(a)	page 357	flail chest
106.	(b)	page 357	flail chest
107.	(e)	page 357	flail chest
108.	(a)	page 358	hemothorax
109.	(a)	page 359	traumatic asphyxia
110.	(d)	page 358	cardiac tamponade
111.	(a)	page 359	tension pneumothorax
112.	(b)	page 37	esophagus
113.	(d)	page 40	solid abdominal organs
114.	(e)	page 40	hollow abdominal organs
115.	(c)	page 41	retraperitoneal
116.	(e)	page 41	pelvic cavity
117.	(a)	page 53	pancreas
118.	(c)	page 55	prostate gland
119.	(a)	page 53	liver
120.	(b)	page 54	kidneys
121.	(c)	page 55	seminal vesicles
122.	(e)	g/d	adrenal glands

PAGE REFERENCE

QUESTION	ANSWER	*Emergency Care* *5th edition*	
123.	(a)	page 53	gallbladder/bile ducts
124.	(b)	page 53	ureters
125.	(e)	g/d	spleen
126.	(a)	page 53	appendix
127.	(d)	page 360	spleen
128.	(d)	page 360	peritoneum
129.	(d)	page 360	peritonitis
130.	(e)	page 360	peritonitis
131.	(b)	page 361	projectile wound
132.	(c)	page 361	abdominal injury
133.	(e)	page 362	treatment of abdominal injury
134.	(e)	page 363	pelvic cavity
135.	(d)	page 363	male genitalia injury
136.	(e)	page 364	penis
137.	(d)	page 364	scrotum
138.	(b)	page 364	prostate gland
139.	(a)	page 364	testicles
140.	(c)	page 364	seminal vesicles
141.	(d)	page 365	vagina
142.	(b)	page 365	vulva
143.	(a)	page 365	ovaries
144.	(e)	page 365	fallopian tubes
145.	(c)	page 365	uterus
146.	(e)	page 366	hernia
147.	(a)	page 436	perineum
148.	(d)	page 437	uterus
149.	(d)	page 437	OB kit
150.	(c)	page 437	fetus
151.	(b)	page 438	cervix
152.	(e)	page 438	umbilical cord
153.	(a)	page 438	amniotic sac
154.	(e)	page 438	fetal circulation
155.	(c)	page 438	labor stages
156.	(b)	page 438	labor stages
157.	(d)	page 438	labor stages
158.	(e)	page 438	labor stages
159.	(a)	page 438	cephalic presentation
160.	(b)	page 438	breech presentation
161.	(c)	page 438	crowning
162.	(c)	page 438	crowning
163.	(b)	page 439	dilation
164.	(d)	page 439	bloody show
165.	(e)	page 439	labor timing
166.	(a)	page 439	labor timing

PAGE REFERENCE

QUESTION	ANSWER	*Emergency Care* 5th edition	
167.	(c)	page 439	false labor pains
168.	(e)	page 439	number of pregnancies
169.	(d)	page 439	bowel movements
170.	(b)	page 440	first pregnancy
171.	(a)	page 440	supine hypotensive syndrome
172.	(d)	page 441	delivery in an automobile
173.	(d)	page 442	delivery
174.	(a)	page 442	delivery
175.	(c)	page 442	delivery
176.	(e)	page 442	newborn care
177.	(a)	page 442	newborn care
178.	(b)	page 442	newborn care
179.	(c)	page 444	APGAR scale
180.	(a)	page 444	APGAR scale
181.	(d)	page 444	APGAR scale
182.	(d)	page 444	APGAR scale
183.	(e)	page 444	newborn care
184.	(c)	page 446	newborn care
185.	(c)	page 446	newborn care
186.	(c)	page 447	postdelivery care
187.	(e)	page 447	afterbirth
188.	(d)	page 447	afterbirth
189.	(c)	page 448	postdelivery care
190.	(a)	page 448	postdelivery care
191.	(c)	page 448	postdelivery care
192.	(d)	page 448	complications of delivery
193.	(b)	page 449	nonbreathing baby
194.	(e)	page 449	nonbreathing baby
195.	(c)	page 450	prolonged delivery
196.	(b)	page 450	prebirth bleeding
197.	(d)	page 451	placenta previa
198.	(b)	page 451	abruptio placentae
199.	(a)	page 451	toxemia of pregnancy
200.	(e)	page 451	eclampsia
201.	(c)	page 451	treatment of toxemia
202.	(c)	page 452	ectopic pregnancy
203.	(b)	page 452	trauma and pregnancy
204.	(e)	page 452	miscarriage
205.	(b)	page 453	ruptured uterus
206.	(e)	page 454	limb presentation
207.	(c)	page 454	abnormal presentation
208.	(c)	page 454	abnormal presentation
209.	(b)	page 455	multiple births
210.	(d)	page 455	premature births

QUESTION	ANSWER	PAGE REFERENCE *Emergency Care* *5th edition*	
211.	(b)	page 461	radiation burns
212.	(a)	page 461	electrical burns
213.	(b)	page 461	burns
214.	(e)	page 461	burns
215.	(c)	page 461	burns
216.	(d)	page 461	burns
217.	(c)	page 461	burns
218.	(c)	page 461	burns
219.	(d)	page 461	burns
220.	(d)	page 462	circumferential burns
221.	(a)	page 463	critical burns
222.	(d)	page 463	rule of nines
223.	(c)	page 463	rule of nines
224.	(e)	page 463	burn treatment
225.	(e)	page 464	burn treatment
226.	(b)	page 465	burn treatment
227.	(c)	page 468	chemical burn treatment
228.	(a)	page 468	smoke inhalation
229.	(a)	page 468	chemicals in the eyes
230.	(c)	page 469	electrical burns
231.	(e)	page 471	radiation burns
232.	(b)	page 471	hazardous materials
233.	(b)	page 475	radiation burn treatment
234.	(c)	page 502	patient communication
235.	(e)	page 507	grief stages
236.	(e)	page 507	grief stages
237.	(b)	page 509	altered level of consciousness
238.	(b)	page 509	restraints
239.	(d)	page 510	suicidal patient
240.	(c)	page 511	rape victim
241.	(e)	page 511	EMT stress
242.	(a)	page 511	EMT stress
243.	(c)	g/d	peristalsis
244.	(b)	g/d	fontanels
245.	(a)	g/d	mediastinum
246.	(b)	g/d	pericardium
247.	(e)	g/d	liver
248.	(c)	g/d	pancreas
249.	(c)	g/d	priapism
250.	(b)	g/d	projectile vomiting

GUIDE TO COMMON MEDICAL ABBREVIATIONS AND SYMBOLS

Many of the following abbreviations were used in this text. For the purpose of self-improvement, this is a more comprehensive list. It contains abbreviations the professional EMT should be familiar with and use on a regular basis. When an abbreviation is based on the Latin or Greek form of a word, the Latin or Greek word is presented in parentheses to improve the EMT's understanding of the origin of the abbreviation.

The appropriate use of upper- and lowercase letters is an important distinction in medical abbreviations. For example: "cc" is the abbreviation for cubic centimeter, whereas "CC" is the abbreviation for chief complaint. And "Ca" is the abbreviation for calcium, whereas "CA" is the abbreviation for cancer.

$\bar{a}$ .... before (*ante*)
AAOX3 .... alert and oriented to person/place/time
abdo .... abdomen
AMA .... against medical advice
AMI .... acute myocardial infarction/heart attack
ASA .... acetylsalicylic acid/aspirin
ASHD .... arteriosclerotic heart disease

BCP .... birth control pills
bid .... twice a day (*bis in die*)
BM .... bowel movement
BS .... breath sounds/blood sugar
BVM .... bag-valve-mask device

$\bar{c}$ .... with (*cum*)
CA .... cancer
CAD .... coronary artery disease
cc .... cubic centimeter
CC .... chief complaint
CHF .... congestive heart failure
cm .... centimeter
CNS .... central nervous system
c/o .... complains of
CO .... carbon monoxide
CO_2 .... carbon dioxide
conx .... conscious
COPD/COLD .... chronic obstructive pulmonary (lung) disease
cp .... chest pain
CSF .... cerebrospinal fluid
CVA .... cerebrovascular accident/stroke

dc ....discontinue
Dx..diagnosis/dislocation

ea ....each
ED ....Emergency Department
EMS ....Emergency Medical Services
EMT ....Emergency Medical Technician
EMT-B ....Emergency Medical Technician—Basic level
EMT-I ....Emergency Medical Technician—Intermediate
EMT-P ....Emergency Medical Technician—Paramedic
ER ....Emergency Room
et ....and (*et*)
ETOH ....alcohol (ethyl alcohol)

FROM ....full range of motion
Fx ....fracture

GI ....gastrointestinal
Gm/gm ....gram
GSW ....gunshot wound
GU ....genitourinary
GYN ....gynecological

HA ....headache
HEENT ....head, ears, eyes, nose, throat
Hx ....history

ICP...intercranial pressure
ICS ....intercostal space

JVD ....jugular vein distention

Kg/kg...kilogram

Ⓛ ....left
lac ....laceration
LBB ....long backboard
LLQ...left lower quadrant
LMP ....last menstrual period
lpm ....liters per minute
LUQ ....left upper quadrant
LOC ....level of consciousness (*not* loss of conx!)

MAST ....military anti-shock trousers
mg ....milligram
MI ....myocardial infarction/heart attack
MICU ....mobile intensive care unit
ml ....milliliter
mm ....millimeter

MOI .... mechanism of injury

n/a .... not applicable
NPO .... nothing by mouth (nothing *per os*)
nc .... nasal cannula
NRB .... nonrebreather mask
NTG .... nitroglycerine
n/v .... nausea and vomiting
n/v/d .... nausea, vomiting, and diarrhea

OB .... obstetrics
OBS .... organic brain syndrome
OD .... overdose/right eye (*occulus dexter*)

$\bar{p}$ .... after (*post*)
PASG .... pneumatic anti-shock garment
PE .... pulmonary embolism
PEARL.. pupils equal and reactive to light
PID .... pelvic inflammatory disease
PNS.. peripheral nervous system
po .... by mouth (*per os*)
prn .... as needed (*pro re nata*)
PTOA .... prior to our arrival
PMH.. past medical history

$\bar{q}$ .... every (*quaque*)
qd .... every day (*quaque die*)
qid .... four times a day (*quarter in die*)

Ⓡ.. right
RBC .... red blood cell
R/O .... rule out
RLQ .... right lower quadrant
RUQ .... right upper quadrant
ROM .... range of motion
Rx .... recipe/prescription

$\bar{s}$ .... without (the Latin *sine* or the French, *sans*)
sc/sq .... subcutaneous
sl .... sublingual
SOB .... shortness of breath
s/s... signs and symptoms
Sx .... symptoms

TIA.. transient ischemic attack/"mini-stroke"
TID .... three times a day (*ter in die*)
trans .... transport

Tx .... treatment (*not trans*)

U/A .... upon arrival
unconx .... unconscious
URI .... upper respiratory infection
UTI .... urinary tract infection

WBC .... white blood cell
w/d .... warm and dry
w/d/pink .... warm, dry, and pink
WNL .... within normal limits

y/o .... years old

COMMON MEDICAL SYMBOLS

Symbol	Meaning	Symbol	Meaning
∿∿∿	approximately	⊕	positive for
△	change	⊖	negative for
>	greater than	Ⓗ	husband
<	less than	Ⓕ	father
♀	female	Ⓜ	mother
♂	male	Ⓦ	wife
×	multiply by	⚬⌐	lying
2°	secondary to	⚵	sitting
		⚤	standing